AMC'S BEST BACKPACKING IN THE
MID-ATLANTIC

A Guide to 30 of the Best Multiday Trips from New York to Virginia

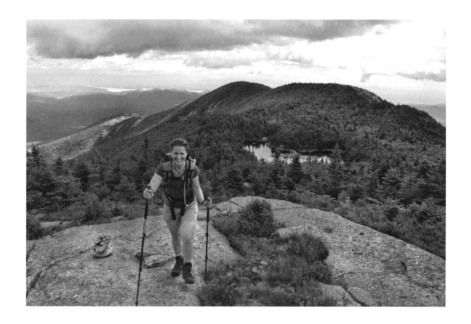

MICHAEL R. MARTIN

T0159363

Appalachian Mountain Club Books
Boston, MA

AMC is a nonprofit organization, and
sales of AMC Books fund our mission of
protecting the Northeast outdoors. If you appreciate our
efforts and would like to become a member or make a donation to AMC,
visit outdoors.org, call 800-372-1758, or contact us at
Appalachian Mountain Club,
5 Joy Street, Boston, MA 02108.
outdoors.org/publications/books

Distributed by The Globe Pequot Press, Guilford, Connecticut.

Front cover photographs: top © Michael Martin, bottom left and right © Jerry and Marcy Monkman,
    bottom center © Tim Messick
Back cover photographs © Michael Martin
Interior photographs © Michael Martin, except on pages 44 and 133 © Brian Horst;
    63 © Max Nemeth; 88 © Christina Louise; 239 © Mike van Wambeke
Maps by Larry Garland © Appalachian Mountain Club
Cover design by Matt Simmons
Interior design by Eric Edstam

Library of Congress Cataloging-in-Publication Data

Martin, Michael R.
  AMC's best backpacking in the Mid-Atlantic : a guide to 30 of the best multi-day trips from New
York to Virginia / Michael R. Martin.
      pages cm.
  ISBN 978-1-934028-86-5 (pbk.)
  1. Backpacking--Middle Atlantic States--Guidebooks. I. Title.
  GV199.42.M52M37 2014
  796.510974--dc23
                    2013048648

The paper used in this publication meets the minimum requirements of the American National
Standard for Information Sciences-Permanence of Paper for Printed Library Materials, ANSI
Z39.48-1984. ∞

Interior pages contain 30% post-consumer recycled fiber.
Cover contains 10% post-consumer recycled fiber.
Printed in the United States of America,
using vegetable-based inks.

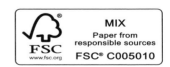

10 9 8 7 6 5 4 3 2 1   13 14 15 16 17

To Laura

LOCATOR MAP

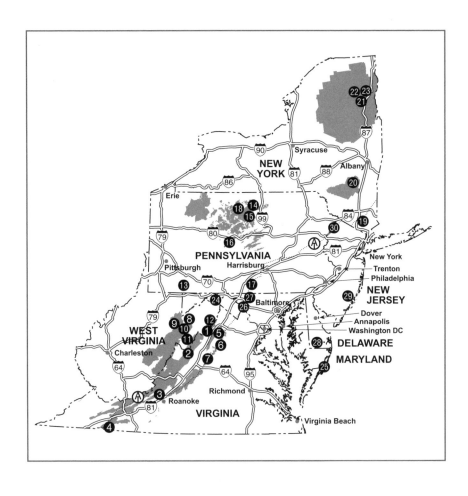

LEGEND

The following icons are used in this book's in-text maps.

————	Backpacking Route
··············	Connecting Trail
════════	Highway
═══════	Improved Road
=========	Unimproved Road (4WD)
— ·· —	Stream
🏠	Lodge, Cabin, or Hut
⬛	Campground
⊏	Shelter
⬛	Tentsite
P	Parking
Ⓐ	Appalachian Trail
▲	Peak or Summit

CONTENTS

Locator Map. iv
Legend v
At-a-Glance Trip Planner. x
Trips by Theme xvi
Preface xix
Acknowledgments xxi
Introduction. xxiii
How to Use This Book. xxv
Where Should I Go Hiking? xxix
Safety, Gear, and Trip Planning. xxxix
Leave No Trace lvii

1 VIRGINIA
Trip 1: Bird's Eye View—Tibbet Knob, George Washington
and Jefferson National Forests 2
Trip 2: Amphibious Landing—Ramseys Draft Wilderness and
Wild Oak Trail, George Washington and Jefferson National Forests 6

Trip 3: Picture Postcard Perfect—Triple Crown, George Washington and Jefferson National Forests 14
Trip 4: High Above the Highlands—Grayson Highlands, George Washington and Jefferson National Forests 24
Trip 5: I Like Big Ridges and I Cannot Lie—Massanutten Ridges, George Washington and Jefferson National Forests 31
Trip 6: The Ragged Edge—Old Rag, Shenandoah National Park 40
Trip 7: Go Big (Run) or Go Home—Big Run, Shenandoah National Park .49

2 WEST VIRGINIA
Trip 8: Hello, Dolly!—Dolly Sods, Monongahela National Forest. 58
Trip 9: Wild, Wonderful. . . and Wet—Otter Creek, Monongahela National Forest 65
Trip 10: (Don't) Get Lost!—Roaring Plains, Monongahela National Forest 72
Trip 11: Carrying Water—North Fork Mountain, Monongahela National Forest 78
Trip 12: King in His Castle—Trout Run Valley, George Washington and Jefferson National Forests 84

3 PENNSYLVANIA
Trip 13: Bear with Me—Bear Run, Bear Run Nature Reserve 92
Trip 14: Rim to Rim to Rim—West Rim Trail, Tioga State Forest 99
Trip 15: Which Way to Munich?—Black Forest Trail, Tiadaghton State Forest. 106
Trip 16: Front and Center—Allegheny Front Trail, Moshannon State Forest 113
Trip 17: Caledonia Dreaming—Pennsylvania Blue Ridge and Rocky Knob, Caledonia State Park and Michaux State Forest. 121
Trip 18: Welcome to the Forest Primeval—Susquehannock Trail System, Susquehannock State Forest 127

4 NEW YORK
Trip 19: Central Park—Bear Mountain, Harriman State Park. 138
Trip 20: A Season in Hell—Devil's Path, Catskill Forest Preserve. 143
Trip 21: The Fjords of New York—Dix Mountain Wilderness Area, Adirondack Forest Preserve 150
Trip 22: Adirondacks the Great—High Peaks Wilderness, Adirondack Forest Preserve 158

Trip 23: Giant Steps—Giant Mountain Wilderness,
Adirondack Forest Preserve 168

5 MARYLAND
Trip 24: Across the River, Through the Woods, and *Under* the Mountain—
C&O Canal, Green Ridge State Forest............................174
Trip 25: Do You Enjoy Long Walks on the Beach?—Assateague,
Assateague Island National Seashore.............................182
Trip 26: View from the Heights—Maryland Blue Ridge and the
Appalachian Trail, Harpers Ferry 190
Trip 27: On the Rocks—Catoctin Trail and the Appalachian Trail,
Gambrill State Park 197

6 NEW JERSEY AND DELAWARE
Trip 28: Beware the Piranha-conda!—Trap Pond, Trap Pond State Park . .208
Trip 29: The Devil Went Down to Jersey—BATONA, Pinelands National
Reserve..213
Trip 30: Hitting the High Notes—Delaware Water Gap and High Point,
Delaware Water Gap National Recreation Area, Stokes State Forest, and
High Point State Park..219

Resources 229
Index..233
About the Author...239
Appalachian Mountain Club 241
AMC in the Mid-Atlantic...243
AMC Book Updates 245

AT-A-GLANCE
TRIP PLANNER

#	Trip	Page	Trailhead Location	Difficulty	Distance and Elevation Gain
	VIRGINIA				
1	Tibbet Knob	2	George Washington and Jefferson National Forests	Moderate	3.1 mi, 1,001 ft
2	Ramseys Draft Wilderness and Wild Oak Trail	6	George Washington and Jefferson National Forests	Challenging	44 mi, 10,461 ft
3	Triple Crown	14	George Washington and Jefferson National Forests	Challenging	34.2 mi, 9,168 ft
4	Grayson Highlands	24	George Washington and Jefferson National Forests	Moderate	26.3 mi, 4,860 ft
5	Massanutten Ridges	31	George Washington and Jefferson National Forests	Epic	67.4 mi, 11,868 ft
6	Old Rag	40	Shenandoah National Park	Challenging	24.2 mi, 7,058 ft
7	Big Run	49	Shenandoah National Park	Strenuous	38.6 mi, 10,149 ft
	WEST VIRGINIA				
8	Dolly Sods	58	Monongahela National Forest	Moderate	24.6 mi, 3,793 ft
9	Otter Creek	65	Monongahela National Forest	Moderate	16 mi, 3,314 ft

Estimated Time	Loop, Car Shuttle, or Out-and-Back	Fee	Dogs Allowed	Dispersed Camping Allowed	Ample Water	Trip Highlights
2 days	Out-and-Back		🐕	⛺	💧	Camp perched above a beautiful Mid-Atlantic valley
3-6 days	Loop		🐕	⛺	💧	Combine a wild creek walk with a beautiful ridge walk
3-4 days	Loop		🐕	⛺	💧	Visit three of the most iconic sights along the AT
2-3 days	Loop	$	🐕	⛺	💧💧	Fine views from the balds of the Grayson Highlands
3-7 days	Loop		🐕	⛺	💧	Epic loop along wild ridges; big views
2-3 days	Loop	$		⛺	💧💧	Scramble to the top of Virginia's most famous peak
2-5 days	Loop	$	🐕	⛺	💧	Explore Shenandoah's dark hollows and high peaks
2-3 days	Loop		🐕	⛺	💧💧	Unique environment of high alpine bogs and meadows
2-3 days	Loop		🐕	⛺	💧💧	Waterfalls and swimming holes in a West Virginia wilderness

#	Trip	Page	Trailhead Location	Difficulty	Distance and Elevation Gain
10	Roaring Plains	72	Monongahela National Forest	Challenging	13.4 mi, 2,587 ft
11	North Fork Mountain	78	Monongahela National Forest	Challenging	23.5 mi, 3,839 ft
12	Trout Run Valley	84	George Washington and Jefferson National Forests	Moderate	27 mi, 5,479 ft
	PENNSYLVANIA				
13	Bear Run	92	Bear Run Nature Reserve	Moderate	14.3 mi, 2,726 ft
14	West Rim Trail	99	Tioga State Forest	Challenging	30 mi, 5,499 ft
15	Black Forest Trail	106	Tiadaghton State Forest	Strenuous	42 mi, 8,807 ft
16	Allegheny Front Trail	113	Moshannon State Forest	Moderate	39.6 mi, 5,470 ft
17	Pennsylvania Blue Ridge and Rocky Knob	121	Caledonia State Park and Michaux State Forest	Moderate	19.6 mi, 3,379 ft
18	Susquehannock Trail System	127	Susquehannock State Forest	Epic	81 mi, 13,050 ft
	NEW YORK				
19	Bear Mountain	138	Harriman State Park	Moderate	11.4 mi, 3,242 ft
20	Devil's Path	143	Catskill Forest Preserve	Strenuous	22.2 mi, 8,686 ft
21	Dix Mountain Wilderness	150	Adirondack Forest Preserve	Challenging	20.1 mi, 7,731 ft

Estimated Time	Loop, Car Shuttle, or Out-and-Back	Fee	Dogs Allowed	Dispersed Camping Allowed	Ample Water	Trip Highlights
2–3 days	Loop		🐕	⛺	💧	Route-find to breathtaking views of the Alleghenies
2–3 days	Car Shuttle		🐕	⛺		Demanding (and dry) ridgeline; a bucket-list must
2–4 days	Loop		🐕	⛺	💧💧	Circumnavigate a valley and visit classic high points
2–3 days	Loop		🐕		💧💧	Woodlands surrounding Fallingwater and the Youghiogheny River gorge
2–4 days	Car Shuttle		🐕	⛺	💧💧	Dramatic route along Pine Creek Gorge, the "Grand Canyon of the East"
2–6 days	Loop		🐕	⛺	💧💧	The state's toughest trail; excellent campsites, big views, swimming, and waterfalls
3–5 days	Loop		🐕	⛺	💧💧	Varied, but gentle, loop
2–3 days	Loop		🐕	⛺	💧💧	A taste of the AT's course across the state
4–10 days	Loop		🐕	⛺	💧💧	Quintessential Allegheny plateau thru-hiking experience; 80 miles of secluded woodlands
2 days	Loop		🐕	⛺	💧	Lovely park just a few minutes away from New York City
2–3 days	Car Shuttle		🐕	⛺	💧	One of the toughest hikes on the East Coast; big views
2–3 days	Loop				💧💧	Four Adirondack 46ers; waterfalls along the Lower Ausable River

#	Trip	Page	Trailhead Location	Difficulty	Distance and Elevation Gain
22	High Peaks Wilderness	158	Adirondack Forest Preserve	Epic	39.7 mi, 12,512 ft
23	Giant Mountain Wilderness	168	Adirondack Forest Preserve	Strenuous	9.9 mi, 5,555 ft
	MARYLAND				
24	C&O Canal	174	Green Ridge State Forest	Moderate	42.3 mi, 4,491 ft
25	Assateague	182	Assateague Island National Seashore	Moderate	27.9 mi, 320 ft
26	Maryland Blue Ridge and the Appalachian Trail	190	Greenbriar State Park	Moderate	24.7 mi, 4,206 ft
27	Catoctin Trail and the Appalachian Trail	197	Gambrill State Park	Strenuous	47.7 mi, 9,047 ft
	NEW JERSEY AND DELAWARE				
28	Trap Pond	208	Trap Pond State Park	Easy	6.8 mi, 192 ft
29	BATONA	213	Pinelands National Reserve	Easy	23.2 mi, 520 ft
30	Delaware Water Gap and High Point	219	Delaware Water Gap National Recreation Area	Challenging	44.1 mi, 7,014 ft

Estimated Time	Loop, Car Shuttle, or Out-and-Back	Fee	Dogs Allowed	Dispersed Camping Allowed	Ample Water	Trip Highlights
4–6 days	Loop	$			●	Eight Adirondack 46ers and unforgettable landmarks
2–3 days	Car Shuttle		🐕		●	An Adirondack traverse, including two 46ers, Giant and Rocky Ridge Mountain Peak
3–5 days	Loop	$	🐕	▲	●	A varied route, including Green Ridge State Forest, the C&O Canal, and the Paw Paw Tunnel
2–3 days	Car Shuttle	$	🐕		●	Pristine, coastal barrier island; camp with the surf pounding nearby
2–3 days	Car Shuttle		🐕		●	Classic AT descent from Weverton Cliffs into Harpers Ferry
3–6 days	Car Shuttle		🐕		●	Picturesque section of the AT with less-often-walked Catoctin Trail
2 days	Loop	$	🐕		●	Lovely coastal wetlands, abundant wildlife, second-growth baldcypress
2–3 days	Car Shuttle		🐕		●	The undeveloped Atlantic coastal forest of the Pine Barrens
3–6 days	Car Shuttle		🐕	▲	●	More than half the AT in New Jersey; summit the state's highest point

TRIPS BY THEME

DAY HIKABLE

1 Tibbet Knob
8 Dolly Sods
9 Otter Creek
10 Roaring Plains
11 North Fork Mountain
13 Bear Run
17 Pennsylvania Blue Ridge
   and Rocky Knob
19 Bear Mountain
20 Devil's Path
23 Giant Mountain Wilderness
25 Assateague
26 Maryland Blue Ridge
   and the Appalachian Trail
28 Trap Pond
29 BATONA

UNUSUAL FORESTS

2 Ramseys Draft Wilderness
   and Wild Oak Trail
8 Dolly Sods
10 Roaring Plains
18 Susquehannock Trail System
28 Trap Pond
29 BATONA

SWIMMING HOLES

6 Old Rag
7 Big Run
9 Otter Creek
15 Black Forest Trail
18 Susquehannock Trail System
22 High Peaks Wilderness
23 Giant Mountain Wilderness
24 C&O Canal

BEST CAMPING SITES

2 Ramseys Draft Wilderness
   and Wild Oak Trail
3 Triple Crown
4 Grayson Highlands
8 Dolly Sods
10 Roaring Plains
11 North Fork Mountain
12 Trout Run Valley
15 Black Forest Trail
18 Susquehannock Trail System
22 High Peaks Wilderness
23 Giant Mountain Wilderness
25 Assateague

WATERFALLS

6 Old Rag
7 Big Run
9 Otter Creek
15 Black Forest Trail
21 Dix Mountain Wilderness
22 High Peaks Wilderness
24 C&O Canal
27 Catoctin Trail and
the Appalachian Trail
30 Delaware Water Gap
and High Point

BIG VIEWS

1 Tibbet Knob
3 Triple Crown
4 Grayson Highlands
5 Massanutten Ridges
6 Old Rag
7 Big Run
8 Dolly Sods
10 Roaring Plains
11 North Fork Mountain
12 Trout Run Valley
14 West Rim Trail
15 Black Forest Trail
19 Bear Mountain
20 Devil's Path
21 Dix Mountain Wilderness
22 High Peaks Wilderness
23 Giant Mountain Wilderness
26 Maryland Blue Ridge and
the Appalachian Trail
27 Catoctin Trail and the
Appalachian Trail
30 Delaware Water Gap
and High Point

LAKES AND PONDS

17 Pennsylvania Blue Ridge
and Rocky Knob
19 Bear Mountain
21 Dix Mountain Wilderness
22 High Peaks Wilderness
23 Giant Mountain Wilderness
28 Trap Pond
29 BATONA
30 Delaware Water Gap
and High Point

MAJOR RIVERS AND OCEAN VIEWS

11 North Fork Mountain
14 West Rim Trail
15 Black Forest Trail
19 Bear Mountain
24 C&O Canal
25 Assateague
26 Maryland Blue Ridge and
the Appalachian Trail
30 Delaware Water Gap
and High Point

FISHING

2 Ramseys Draft Wilderness and
Wild Oak Trail
7 Big Run
9 Otter Creek
12 Trout Run Valley
18 Susquehannock Trail System
22 High Peaks Wilderness
24 C&O Canal
25 Assateague
28 Trap Pond

WILDFLOWERS

4 Grayson Highlands
6 Old Rag
7 Big Run
8 Dolly Sods
10 Roaring Plains
18 Susquehannock Trail System
24 C&O Canal
30 Delaware Water Gap
   and High Point

GOOD FOR KIDS

1 Tibbet Knob
9 Otter Creek
13 Bear Run
14 West Rim Trail
17 Pennsylvania Blue Ridge
   and Rocky Knob
19 Bear Mountain
25 Assateague
26 Maryland Blue Ridge and
   the Appalachian Trail
28 Trap Pond

EPIC ADVENTURES

5 Massanutten Ridges
18 Susquehannock Trail System
22 High Peaks Wilderness

LESS TRAVELED

2 Ramseys Draft Wilderness
   and Wild Oak Trail
5 Massanutten Ridges
18 Susquehannock Trail System
24 C&O Canal
25 Assateague
27 Catoctin Trail and
   the Appalachian Trail
29 BATONA

AUTHOR'S FAVORITES

3 Triple Crown
4 Grayson Highlands
5 Massanutten Ridges
6 Old Rag
10 Roaring Plains
12 Trout Run Valley
15 Black Forest Trail
18 Susquehannock Trail System
21 Dix Mountain Wilderness
22 High Peaks Wilderness
23 Giant Mountain Wilderness
25 Assateague
30 Delaware Water Gap
   to High Point

PREFACE

ABOUT FIVE YEARS AGO, I MOVED TO WASHINGTON, D.C., FROM AUSTIN, TEXAS. As I drove my rental truck north on I-81 on a cold January morning, I marveled at the mountains. To the east, the fabled Blue Ridge was misty and white. To the west, the Alleghenies marched away into the dusk, endlessly.

I had been backpacking since I was a child, but as a Texan, that often meant driving long distances to northern New Mexico, southern Colorado, or the Ozarks. All very fine places, to be sure, but the drives were difficult. I had only been in the D.C. area for a few months before I was spending every weekend hiking or backpacking. I was addicted.

You may be surprised by the wildness of the Mid-Atlantic, as it is one of the most populous regions of the country. It has never ceased to amaze me what great hiking could be had only an hour or two from the Capital Beltway. Even as my range extended to Pennsylvania, New Jersey, and New York, I still haven't done every hike I want to do in the Shenandoah!

This book is a blueprint for exploring this magnificent region of the country, with all its ridges and hollows, all its wonder and beauty. When we titled this book the *Best of Backpacking in the Mid-Atlantic*, we meant it: this guide is intended to be a grand tour of the region's highlights, a top 30 list of Mother Nature's greatest hits.

This book is also an introduction to the great pastime of backpacking. Did I say "pastime"? Well, it's more like a lifestyle. Not only will you find a comprehensive introduction to the equipment you need, but you can gain skill on easier trips listed early in each chapter before progressing on to the more challenging trips.

I hope you enjoy this book at least half as much as I enjoyed writing it. By the time you read this preface, I hope to be out working on a new list of trails. Perhaps it will be called *The 30 Next Best Backpacking Trips in the Mid-Atlantic*. I hope I see you out there.

ACKNOWLEDGMENTS

IN WRITING THIS BOOK, MY DEBTS ARE MANY AND DEEP. First and foremost, I want to thank AMC and the books staff, who helped turn this somewhat misshapen sow's ear into a silk purse. Special thanks to Victoria Sandbrook Flynn, who stepped into the task of editing this book with great vigor and calm. I would also be remiss in not thanking the many forestry personnel and trail clubs who lent their expertise to my work, and helped me get around their necks of the woods.

I owe much gratitude to my many comrades at the D.C. Ultra-Light Backpacking Meet Up. Their willingness to grab their gear and go, no matter how short the notice, unpromising the weather, or insane the adventure, has meant that I did virtually none of these trips alone and often enjoyed plentiful and pleasurable company.

Those DC ULers who offered me aid, advice, and encouragement along the way are too numerous to list, but I want to thank those who kept me company on the trail: Mike Van Wambeke (Eeyore), Doug Wolf, Holger Pflicke, Andrew Mendolia (Hang Glider), Shelby Peterson (Shamrock), Sharon Grant (Macgyver), Dan Fisher (Heavy D), John Callahan, Ben Weaver (Unicorn Dust), Mark Anderson (Mountain Slayer), Miles Barger (The Most Interesting Man in America), Alison Benson (Pretty Good Cover Girl), Mike Korin (LaBamba), Joffrey Peters (Beast Mode), Christy Sappenfield (Tenderfoot), Denise Murray (Twinkle Toes), Katie Hoyt, Christine Eichinger (Her Majesty), Will Fink, Jake Lloyd, Steve Kerr, Chris Harbert, Abby Lindsay, Jimmy "Jinn" Jinn, Carrie Price (Giggles), Anna Oberlander (Pancakes), Amber Thomas, Jasmine Naifund, Andrew Schloeffel, Libby Knight (Short Fuse), Lindsay Kuhn, Kingsley Chan, Michael Dodson, Carolyn Gernand (Virtual Slug), Evan Lepore, Leia Garcia, Reid Mueller, Chris Moran, Michael MacBryde, Peter Silverman (Fiber One), Doug Swiatocha, Brett Kuhnert, George Davis, Travis Warren, Matt Turbyfill, Noam Fine, David Schrock, Noah Osner, Amos

Swogger, George Lambert, John Lambert, and Giuseppe Battaglia. When I headed down the wrong trail, they were always there to point me in the right direction, or call in Big Al for a rescue mission.

A few special shout-outs are in order. To Evan McCarthy, who started it all. To Ryan Shauers, who kept it all going. To Brian Horst (B~~~), who has helped me run it. To Carrie Graff (Booty-Less), who came to my aid when I was pondering the trips in New York. Not only did she lend her expertise, but also she packed her backpack and hit the road with me for two weeks. I hope she bagged some of her dream peaks along the way! To Max Nemeth (Yeti), who has taught me more about backpacking than anyone else, while using the fewest words. To Jen Adach (Shuttle), my friend and coconspirator, who saw me through the whole endeavor.

In thinking about the contributions of all these wonderful people and great backpackers over the course of writing this book, I can't escape concluding what a collective process it has been. Though there's a great deal of backpacking going on in the Mid-Atlantic, this is the first book to unite all the best backpacking trips in the region. That's an amazing fact. Many of the trips in this book are classics, well trod and well known. But there are also many trips that my backpacking friends have stitched together from bits and pieces of famous trails, always looking to add a few extra miles or find an appealing new campsite. Truly, this is their book as much as mine—I'm sure many of them will recognize themselves in its pages.

To my old trail dog Fritz, who ran his last mile on these trips. I miss him greatly.

To my parents, who imparted to me my love of the outdoors on those long vacations out west in the battered 1973 International pickup truck, with the camper on the back. They couldn't have guessed that taking me back to the Grand Canyon (because I wanted to get to the bottom) would one day result in this book.

And, finally and most importantly, to Laura (Black and Blue), who certainly didn't know what she was getting into when she married a backpacker. Writing a book like this one is a long journey away from home. Thank you for your patience, sympathy, and love on the homeward trip and for understanding when I took just one more trip to get the details right. I look forward to the many dawns we'll enjoy together.

INTRODUCTION

MUCH OF MY ENERGY IN WRITING THIS BOOK has gone into making it useful to backpackers of all levels of ability and inclinations. If you get ten backpackers together and ask them for the best way to walk a certain trail, you're likely to get twelve to fourteen answers. I am, by inclination, rather an athletic hiker: I like to wake up early, walk swiftly all day, and pitch camp in the twilight. But I know that many backpackers would regard my tendency to rush by a plant of interest or a captivating photographic moment with a measure of horror. Many others would be appalled to see me pass up an opportunity for a beautiful late afternoon campsite only to end up pitching in a bramble patch far from any water source an hour after sunset. Others would definitely look down their noses at how spartan my backcountry kitchen is.

The great commandment of backpacking is, as you may know, "Hike your own hike." Take my hike descriptions and adapt them to your own inclinations. You can walk them exactly as they're written, but more slowly, so that you can take the time to set up for a great photograph, bring your binoculars and go birding, or even bait a fishing pole. You also can walk them completely differently, perhaps breaking them up into affairs of several weekends. In fact, each hike description has an "Other Options" section where I include some suggestions for how the trip could be adapted to suit other backpacking tastes. If you start playing with these options, you'll quickly find that this is not a book of 30 trips, but more like 90! Talk about value for your money.

.

HOW TO USE THIS BOOK

FOR THE PURPOSES OF THIS BOOK, the Mid-Atlantic is divided into five geographic areas—Virginia, West Virginia, Pennsylvania, New York, Maryland, and the Coastal Mid-Atlantic, which includes Delaware and New Jersey. Trips are listed separately within each region. Maps at the beginning of each section help you identify the trip location.

If you're new to backpacking, start your Mid-Atlantic adventures with easy trips. These hikes feature lower mileage, easier terrain, and great rewards for just a few miles of walking. For your very first trip, consider Tibbet Knob (Trip 1) or Trap Pond (Trip 28). Once you're comfortable spending a night outdoors, continue to build skill and expertise with Otter Creek, West Virginia (Trip 9); Bear Run, Pennsylvania (Trip 13); Pennsylvania Blue Ridge and Rocky Knob (Trip 17); and Maryland Blue Ridge and the Appalachian Trail (Trip 26). Beginner backpackers who work through these four trips will come away with a good overview of the region and solid set of basic backpacking skills. In short, you'd no longer be a beginner.

As an intermediate backpacker, keep expanding your range by doing trips like Grayson Highlands, Virginia (Trip 4); Dolly Sods, West Virginia (Trip 8); North Fork Mountain, West Virginia (Trip 11); Trout Run, West Virginia (Trip 12); West Rim, Pennsylvania (Trip 14); and Harriman State Park, New York (Trip 19). By the time you're ready to backpack around the Allegheny Front Trail in Pennsylvania (Trip 16), you're in the big leagues and you can approach any trip in this book.

If you're new to the Mid-Atlantic outdoors, refer to the Introduction for information on geography and seasonality. Readers should take the time to familiarize themselves with the Safety, Gear, and Trip Planning and Leave No Trace sections before setting out. If you're looking for a specific feature, consult the Trips by Theme section. Otherwise, flip through this guide page by page and evaluate each adventure based on the standard information provided.

BACKPACKING TRIPS

Each trip description uses a standard template that makes it easy to compare trips, no matter their differences. This template is divided into two parts: the Header and the Hike Description.

THE HEADER

Title. A fun and often fanciful title to capture your imagination. You won't find this title on maps, signs, or anywhere else except this book.

Icons. Once you settle on a destination and turn to a trip in this guide, you will find a series of icons that indicate whether dogs may hike with you, fees are charged, water is plentiful, and primitive backcountry camping is allowed along the route.

Location. Identifies the area or specific destination the hike visits.

Highlights. What makes the trip special, unique, and impossible to resist.

Distance. The total mileage of the hike, as determined by a handheld Global Positioning System (GPS) unit and authoritative references. For point-to-point hikes, the one-way distance is listed.

Total Elevation Gain/Loss. The amount of climbing and descending on the hike, measured in vertical feet. Total gain/loss can be (and usually is) much greater than the difference between the hike's lowest and highest points. The elevation gain is calculated from measurements and information from U.S. Geological Survey (USGS) topographic maps, landowner maps, and Google Earth.

Trip Length. The number of days recommended to complete the trip. A range of days is usually listed; that range is dependent on your pace. The lower value represents timing for an experienced and fast hiker, while the upper value estimates a more moderate speed for an intermediate backpacker. You should be aware of your physical capabilities and limitations when selecting a hike. A reasonably fit hiker can average 2–3 MPH over flat or gradual descents, 1–2 MPH on gradual climbs, and just 1 MPH on the steepest ascents. You may have to adjust the trip length based on your pace and predilection for walking long days.

Difficulty. The book uses a five-point difficulty rating system:

Easy. Short and level, these hikes can be done by nearly anybody and have less than 500 feet of elevation gain.

Moderate. Longer hikes with 500–3,000 feet of total elevation gain per day along good, easy-to-follow trails. Suitable for any reasonably fit hiker.

Challenging. Difficult hikes with 1,000–3,000 feet of elevation gain per day on more challenging trails. Good fitness required.

Strenuous. A very challenging hike involving considerable elevation gain and loss on difficult trails. Higher mileage can also increase the difficulty to this rating.

Epic. Extended adventures with considerable and constant elevation gain and loss, often in remote regions on challenging trails. Experienced backpackers only.

The ratings are based on my experiences, and they are my estimates of what the average hiker will experience. You may find them to be easier or more difficult than stated. Remember that you can always make a tough trip a little easier by going slower or make an easy trip tougher by speeding up or visiting during inclement weather.

Recommended Maps and Other Resources. No pains have been spared to produce fine-looking maps in this book, and some of the trips could be completed using only the maps included. You'll enjoy yourself more and have greater opportunities for learning about backcountry navigation if you pair a photocopy of the trip map from this book with a topographic map of the area. For every trip listed, the relevant USGS quadrants have been provided, along with names of the best maps of the area. Having a detailed topographic map is essential for your safety if you find yourself having to navigate in the backcountry; a map printed in a book should not replace a highly detailed, expert reference.

Other books and resources that aided in the writing of this book are also listed. These are well worth checking out if, like many hikers, you enjoy reading as much as you can about a trail before you head out the door.

HIKE DESCRIPTION

The hike description is broken down into seven main sections:

Hike Overview

A general overview of the trip, discussing highlights and the broad characteristics of the route. In this section I address which level of backpacker will find this trip the most rewarding.

Overnight Options

A detailed description of established campsites, shelters, lean-tos, backcountry campsites, and other overnight options, including mileages, latitude and longitude noted in degree decimal format, natural setting, and amenities. Information about reservations and beating the crowds is included in this section.

How To Reach the Trailhead

Concise driving directions to the trailhead, including the latitude and longitude of the trailhead. This book assumes that you have a basic highway map of the Mid-Atlantic. Every car's odometer is a little different, so please note that mileages may vary slightly in your vehicle.

Hike Description

A detailed narrative of the hike. Parenthetical notations such as (1.5/3,240) are included at relevant points to denote the distance traveled from the trailhead, in miles (1.5) and the elevation in feet at that point (3,240). Occasional notations of peaks are also noted parenthetically, such as Mount Marcy (5,344). Summits along the trail also include latitude and longitude coordinates for reference, such as Tibbet Knob (1.6/2,930/38° 54.8560' N, 78° 42.2994' W).

Other Options

Look to these sections for ways to shorten a hike, break it up into more manageable sections, add more challenges, or extend the hike to get in a few more miles.

Nearby

After a few nights sleeping on the ground, you may find yourself in need of a good restaurant or pub. This section will point you in the right direction after you return to the trailhead.

Additional Information

Addresses, telephone numbers, and websites for additional sources of information about the trail.

WHERE SHOULD I GO HIKING?

MID-ATLANTIC GEOGRAPHY AND TOPOGRAPHY

In general, the Mid-Atlantic is defined by a relatively flat coastal plain where the majority of the population lives (D.C., Baltimore, Philadelphia, and New York) and the Appalachian Mountain system rising to the west in a series of dramatic ridges that tend to run north–south. In between is an area of low, rolling hills known as the Piedmont.

Virginia (Trips 1–7)

Virginia typifies this pattern. From the populous coastal plains regions in the east, the state becomes increasingly mountainous as you move farther west. Beyond the hills of the Piedmont rises the Blue Ridge, almost as if it were the state's backbone. Along this ridgeline runs the Appalachian Trail (AT). With Shenandoah National Park located along this ridge, you'll find some of the best hiking in Virginia in these mountains (Trips 2, 3, 4, 5 and 6).

But of course there is more to Virginia than a single ridge, even if it is picturesque. If you stand atop Shenandoah's tallest peak, Hawksbill Mountain (4,050), you'll be treated to a 360-degree view of the area's topography. Looking west, you'll see the lower, but very distinct, ridges of Massanutten Mountain (hike these on Trip 5) and beyond them the ridgelines of the Alleghenies. These ridge and valley systems form the border with West Virginia, each north-and-south line separated from the next by deep and fertile agricultural valleys. Several of the trips in this book will take you to these wilder ridges, comparatively far from the more easily reached Blue Ridge.

This topography will shape how you'll hike. In many cases, a typical trip will start with climbing one of these ridges. Once you've gained the ridge, though, you'll often enjoy fairly easy walking, with the occasional descent into a hollow or gap and the occasional ascent to a peak.

Another curiosity of Virginia is that it has virtually no natural lakes, since the glaciers that formed the northern lakes didn't reach so far south. If you see a lake or a pond, it is almost certainly artificially constructed.

West Virginia (Trips 8–12)

Except for a few river valleys, little land in West Virginia is flat. In sharp contrast with the coastal plain, piedmont, and ridge system in Virginia and Maryland, West Virginia is comparatively a crumpled mass of ridges with fairly narrow valleys in between. The border itself is a ridgeline, and you'll feel that you're passing over one mountain after another as you drive to the trailheads in this book. You'll sense that this is wilder and more isolated country. After you've hiked here a bit, you won't be surprised to learn that when the AT was threatened by property rights issues in the 1960s, the Tuscarora Trail was constructed to bypass northern Virginia and Maryland and reroute the AT through wilder West Virginia to Pennsylvania.

Many of the trips in this book are set up to take advantage of this topography, either following ridges and hunting for big views (like Trips 10 and 12) or exploring the deep hollows of Otter Creek (Trip 9).

A perennial favorite for backpackers, Dolly Sods (Trip 8) is located in a unique environment in the region. With an average altitude of 2,700 feet, Dolly Sods is the highest plateau in the United States east of the Mississippi River. With its wind-stunted trees, its big open views of the surrounding mountains, and its bogs, it is more characteristic of a landscape you might expect to see in Canada. Backpackers have not really experienced all the region has to offer until they have wandered the trails of Dolly Sods.

Pennsylvania (Trips 13–18)

Pennsylvania is known as the "Keystone State" because it sits at a geographical (and cultural) crossroads between the south and New York and New England, as well as between the East and the Midwest. But it is also interesting in topographical terms.

While the ridge and valley system that characterizes the southern states also crisscrosses Pennsylvania from the south-central part of the state to the northeast, much of the central section of the country is dominated by the Allegheny Plateau, a land feature so deeply cut by streams and rivers that it often seems mountainous, even though it isn't truly a mountain range.

While the AT sticks to the southern ridges and heads to the New Jersey border (Trip 17), the best hiking in Pennsylvania is to be found in the Allegheny Plateau (Trips 14, 15, 16, and 18). For the hiker, this comparatively wild and unsettled land will feel quite different. You may never ascend from a trailhead as dramatically as you might in Virginia. Instead, you'll often find yourself parking on the plateau, descending deep into hollows, and then climbing back out of them. Although the mountains will not seem as high as Virginia or New York, you'll find the hiking challenging.

The plateau and hollow topography means that Pennsylvania does not always abound in great views, but this book will guide you to the best of them. From the vistas on Black Forest Trail, you'll gain a strong sense of how waterways like Pine Creek have carved their way into the bones of this country. Likewise, the views from the Allegheny Front will enable you to peer southward off the plateau toward the Mason-Dixon Line.

New York (Trips 19–23)

If Pennsylvania is a "keystone," then the Empire State is the capstone for the territory covered in this book. Home to fascinating geography, New York is also where the ridge and valley system that characterizes so much of the region comes to an end, south of the Mohawk River and west of the Hudson.

There are three distinct mountain ranges in New York. The first and easternmost is an extension of the Blue Ridge that enters New York from New Jersey and arcs across the state just north of New York City. As you stand atop Bear Mountain, along the Hudson River, and in Harriman State Park, you'll gain a good sense of these mountains and of the terrain the AT crosses through on its way to New England (Trip 19).

An extension of the Allegheny Plateau that so dominates Pennsylvania, the Catskills and the Shawangunk mountains extend into the center of the state and offer backpackers excellent opportunities fairly near the cities. You'll know you're in the Catskills when you have "two rocks for every dirt." As you walk along the spine of peaks above 3,500 feet that form the Devil's Path, you'll gain a keen appreciation for the ruggedness of this topography (Trip 20).

As the crown jewel of backpacking in New York, the Adirondacks are the third and most impressive chain of mountains in New York, and the largest park in the contiguous United States. They are also geologically distinct. Instead of the ridge-and-valley structure that typifies much of the Mid-Atlantic, the Adirondacks are formed by uplift, forming a dome more than 150 miles wide. As you stand on Mount Colvin and peer into the abyss of Lower Ausable Lake, you'll be able to picture the forces of erosion that have molded these mountains into their current steep and forbidding form (Trip 21). If you are seduced by the siren song of climbing all 46 peaks over 4,000 feet—including the state's high point, Mount Marcy (5,344)—you'll be off to a good start by completing the trips in this book. No fewer than fourteen of the Adirondacks' highest peaks (the 46ers) are covered in these routes (Trips 21, 22, and 23). Many 46ers offer you stunning 360-degree views of this vast wilderness.

New York is also distinct in that, because the state saw extensive glaciation, it offers backpackers the chance to walk along lakeshores. Few lakeshore hikes will rival the walk along Lake Colden and Avalanche Lake (Trip 22).

Maryland (Trips 24–27)

Although the vast majority of the population and landmass of Maryland is within the coastal plain, the state shares geographic features with its neighbor, Virginia. If your eye follows the "arm" of Maryland from Baltimore west to Ohio, you'll cross all the same ridges that give Virginia its unique topography—the Blue Ridge, the valley and ridge system, and the Alleghenies in the far west.

The hiker's interest in Maryland will naturally center on the Blue Ridge as it enters the state from Harpers Ferry in the south and makes for Pennsylvania in the north. This line, of course, is also followed by the Appalachian Trail, which runs for about 41 miles through Maryland. If you hike Trips 26 and 27, you'll have done about 35 of these 41 miles. Trip 27 will also take you to the nearby Catoctin Mountain system, which is also very scenic and features views looking out over the Piedmont toward Baltimore. On Trip 26, pay particular attention to the view from White Rocks. On a clear day looking south toward the Virginia ridges, you'll easily appreciate just how challenging is the AT's course.

Further west, in Maryland's "arm," backpackers will enjoy more isolation hiking in Green Ridge State Forest along a route that combines ridge and hollow-walking in the Alleghenies with a tour of the C&O Canal and the Paw Paw Tunnel (Trip 24).

The fourth and final trip in Maryland takes place on Assateague Island, a barrier island that is ceaselessly being shaped and reshaped by the wind and the waves. This beach environment is unlike any other featured in this book (Trip 25).

New Jersey and Delaware (Trips 28–30)

The coastal plains dominate Delaware and much of New Jersey; in fact, Delaware sits entirely on the Delmarva Peninsula, which it shares in part with Maryland. Although Delaware cannot boast the mountainous Appalachian terrain that characterizes so much of the Mid-Atlantic, a visit to Trap Pond will enable a backpacker to catch a glimpse of what these coastal wetlands looked like before they were settled (Trip 28).

New Jersey is also home to a unique environment for backpacking—the Pine Barrens. This section of the coastal plains is almost entirely flat. Its sandy, acidic soil made farming difficult; as a result, the area was never settled extensively. A variety of interesting flora may be found there, including orchids and carnivorous plants. It's also the home of the fabled Jersey Devil and the site of a memorable *Sopranos* episode (Trip 29).

New Jersey's northwestern corner, however, is highly reminiscent of Virginia. As your eye moves from the southeastern corner of the state northwesterly across the map, you'll see the familiar layering of piedmont, highland, valley and ridges, and eventually the ridgeline of the Kittatinny Mountains. The Kittatinnies are effectively cousins to the ridgelines running northeasterly throughout Pennsylvania.

This dramatic ridge is home to the Appalachian Trail as it darts up to the New York State line before heading east. Trip 30 begins at the Delaware Water Gap, where the Delaware River has cut its way through these mountainous barriers on its path to the sea, and follows the AT north to High Point, New Jersey.

BEATING THE CROWDS

It may seem like a strange thing to say, but despite the fact that 20 percent of the population of the United States lives in the Mid-Atlantic, you won't have any difficulty finding solitude in its backcountry. There are a few areas where you can anticipate Yosemite-like crowds. Old Rag and the central district of the Shenandoah, Mount Marcy, and the stretch of the Appalachian Trail through Maryland see a great deal of traffic on a nice spring day. If you go a little off-season or get a nice early-morning start, even those areas can be blissfully quiet. Weekday visits will also help you enjoy the tranquility of nature.

The wildness and solitude of the region will only deepen as you drive a little farther from the big cities. Reach Massanutten Mountain and you'll see only the occasional other hiker or backpacker. Drive farther, to the Alleghenies or the wilds of Potter County, Pennsylvania, and you might very well find yourself entirely alone. Even though you will see evidence of humankind (road crossings, telecommunications relays, etc.), there are so many trails for backpackers to enjoy that you may find yourself walking entire loops without seeing another soul. See the Trips by Theme section for some of the least traveled routes in the book.

If you really want solitude, you can always head out when the weather looks less than ideal. Though this isn't fun for everyone, Mother Nature can be at her most striking when she is hitting you with some unpleasant weather. And, of course, the absence of fair-weather hikers means that you'll have the trail to yourself. Just be prepared for the elements.

It should also be noted that the Appalachian Trail, with its annual migration of thru-hikers, plays a role in many of the trips in this book. Thru-hikers will be present on the trail, predominantly headed north, through spring and summer. Most hikers spend April, May, or June along the Appalachian Trail in Virginia. They try to make it north of Harpers Ferry and through the Mid-Atlantic before the heat sets in during early summer. It's fine to be out on the trail while the thru-hikers are coming by. In fact, plan a little trail magic (spontaneous acts of generosity toward thru-hikers). Do be aware, however, that the shelters are really for their use. You're only going out for a night or two, so carry your tent.

THE MID-ATLANTIC, SEASON BY SEASON

Because this is three-season guide, this section covers the nine months in the Mid-Atlantic when you can reasonably expect to venture into the backcountry and enjoy good weather—March through November. Please note that the Mid-Atlantic is a big place, and that winter in the Adirondacks starts sooner than in southwest Virginia. In upstate New York, consider winter as occurring from November through March, and probably think of October and April as shoulder-season weather.

It's possible to do some of the trips in this book in winter. The book, however, does not discuss how snow or ice affects these trips, nor does it discuss the range of skills or equipment you need for winter camping and backpacking. Make sure you seek out those skills before you head out when snow is in the air. Going with a veteran winter camper is the best way to learn.

Climatologically speaking, there are really two climates in the region. New York, Pennsylvania, and northern New Jersey have short and warm summers, while the rest of the region experiences long, hot, and humid summers with short, mild winters.

March. While in most years you'll still be dealing with winter conditions in Pennsylvania and New York, March can already be excellent backpacking weather in the lower reaches of the region. Some of the trips in this book are even best walked in early spring, such as Assateague (Trip 25), where you'll have solitude along the beaches and no insects. Do pay attention to the first humid-feeling day in Virginia, as that's usually a sign that the insects are about to hatch. Don't forget your headnet. When backpacking in March, be aware that the weather can turn wintery in a flash. Be prepared for a sudden freeze and have an extra layer in your pack.

April. Everywhere except the Adirondacks, spring will be in full bloom and backpacking season will be on. A wonderful month for backpacking: it's really tough to go wrong.

May. Perhaps the best spring month for backpacking throughout the region. Wildflowers will be in bloom, but of course it is also time for the insects. Practice good tick awareness throughout spring. Temperatures can periodically become humid and summery. Memorial Day is an excellent time to go backpacking, but conditions can sometimes become jungle-like.

June. In the south, June is early summer, but the temperatures are not warm enough to make backpacking miserable—you can still have some well-nigh perfect backpacking weather.

July and August. Unless you like the heat, these will be some of the toughest months of the year for backpacking. In the south, the heat and humidity can really become quite unbearable, so pick one of the swimming hole trips (Trips 2, 6, 7, 9, 15, 18, 18, 20, 22, 23, and 24) or perhaps seek out one of the higher elevation hikes in West Virginia (Trips 8 and 11). Combining a leisurely trip into Harpers Ferry with a tubing trip down the Potomac is also great fun (Trip 26). Be prepared to dial back the mileage in the heat, walk in the mornings and the evenings, and be sure to hydrate. These months are also a good time to drive north and visit New York. Bagging a few 46ers may be in order (Trips 21, 22, and 23).

September. For Virginia, West Virginia, Maryland, and portions of Pennsylvania, September remains a summer month, though the temperatures will be a bit more moderate, making it a considerably better time to backpack. Autumn will be setting in farther north, making it an excellent time to head to the Catskills or the Adirondacks. Trips like the traverse of the Giant Mountain Wilderness (Trip 23) or the circumnavigation of Trout Run Valley (Trip 2) might even come close to rivaling New England's fall foliage.

October. This is one of the most splendid months for backpacking in the southern Appalachians. The temperatures will be cool and crisp, the foliage will be marching down the Blue Ridge and toward the Smokies, and the winter views will be just starting to open out. If you head at all north, you should be prepared for cold, but generally three-season conditions will last throughout the month. Go out every weekend and watch the leaves modulate their colors.

November. By November, winter has started to settle in throughout most of the northern reaches of the Mid-Atlantic, so the New York trips will be under the pall of winter. In most of the rest of the region, however, you're effectively getting an extra month of good, solid, three-season hiking weather. The leaves will be off the trees, so the views will open out. You should plan on this being shoulder-season weather—warmer clothes and a bag liner might be in order. Nighttime temperatures could dip below freezing, and you could see some wintery precipitation. Do keep your eye on the weather report.

NATURAL HISTORY OF THE MID-ATLANTIC

From the shores of Assateague to the summit of Mount Marcy, the Mid-Atlantic displays a rich variety of forest types that are notable for their biological diversity—158 different species of trees may be found here. These forests are the remnants of a vast and ancient forest that once spread across much of North America. Heavily logged during the settling of the United States, almost all of these forests are composed of second-growth trees that are less than a century old.

Barrier islands. Along the sandy shoreline, only a few varieties of grasses are able to prosper in the surf, spray, and wind. As you move inland, more plants thrive in the dunes. Farther inland, as backpackers will note on the bay side of Assateague (Trip 25), a maritime forest grows, made up of loblolly pine, sweetgum, post oak, red maple, and black cherry.

Wetlands. Throughout the coastal plain, one may find wetlands where baldcypress and red maple withstand frequent flooding. Backpackers can experience this environment by visiting Trap Pond (Trip 28). The Pine Barrens (Trip 29) is also a coastal wetland, though it is unique due to its exceptionally acidic soil.

Piedmont forests. Less dry than the forests of the ridge and valley system, these forests are dominated by oaks and hickories. Backpackers will find these sorts of forests along the Maryland AT (Trips 26 and 27), as well as the eastward face of the Shenandoah.

Northern hardwood forest. A variety of northern hardwood forests occur throughout the region. On the Allegheny Plateau, sugar maple, basswood, yellow birch, black birch, American beech, and black cherry dominate. Hikers might visit these forests while backpacking the West Rim and Black Forest trails (Trips 14 and 15). In the warmer ridge and valley system in Virginia, oaks dominate, as one would observe in the Shenandoah or the Massanuttens (Trips 5, 6, and 7). In the Adirondacks, these types of forests yield to balsam fir and black spruce as the elevation rises. Hikers will note dwarfed and contorted forests, known as "krummholz," as they approach tree line (Trips 21, 22, and 23).

Boreal forest. On the highest points of the Allegheny Plateau, red spruce dominate, along with hardwood trees such as maple, yellow birch, American beech, and black cherry. Visitors to areas such as Dolly Sods (Trip 8) or Roaring Plains (Trip 10) will find that they commonly encounter bogs, such as along Dobbin Grade.

Appalachian balds. Balds are mountain summits or crests that would ordinarily be covered by forests, but instead are open and covered by grasses or shrubs. Backpackers walking over the balds in the Grayson Highlands of southwest Virginia will be able enjoy vistas taking in the mountains of Tennessee and North Carolina (Trip 4).

Alpine zone. On eleven peaks above 4,000 feet in the Adirondacks, the year-round climate becomes too harsh to support trees, and a variety of lichens and mosses that one would expect to find much farther north have taken hold. Such environments are, of course, beautiful to hike through, but they are easily damaged by hikers. Stay on the trails and avoid stepping on the vegetation. Hikers will visit several peaks with such environments in the Adirondacks (Trips 21, 22, and 23).

For additional information on the forest types of the Mid-Atlantic, the studious backpacker should consult Mark Garland's *Watching Nature: A Mid-Atlantic Natural History*, to which my short discussion is greatly indebted.

CONSERVATION OF THE MID-ATLANTIC

The diverse ecosystems and dense population centers of the Mid-Atlantic region bring with them a range of environmental concerns. Logging, mining, water diversion, and agriculture all took their toll on the region's natural resources long before conservation efforts began; today, air and water pollution, invasive species, forest fragmentation, and overuse continue to factor into the health of the Mid-Atlantic's wild areas.

Possibly the most often discussed issues in the Mid-Atlantic (at the time of publication) are natural gas drilling and hydraulic fracturing, or "fracking," on conserved land. While many public forests and parks are protected from the encroachment of industry, the rights to minerals below the surface are often privately owned; restricting private companies from developing natural gas wells on the surface would also restrict their access to the gas they own. Opponents, however, highlight the potential risk of groundwater contamination and spills—both particularly dangerous for already fragile protected land. Beyond the impact of the drilling itself, infrastructure for these operations—from roads to pipelines to containment ponds—must be built, increasing both the potential footprint and the likelihood of impact on trails and viewsheds.

Drilling has already begun on public lands in some states. In Pennsylvania, you may encounter evidence of drilling on the West Rim Trail (Trip 14), the

Allegheny Front Trail (Trip 16), and on the Susquehannock Trail System (Trip 18). Though drilling is prevalent in West Virginia and is planned in Maryland and New York, it does not currently impact the trips in this book. To date, at least one major drilling debate continues in the Mid-Atlantic: as of November, 2013, the U.S. Forest Service had not yet released a decision in the heated battle over drilling rights in George Washington and Jefferson National Forests in Virginia and West Virginia.

Maps of oil and gas wells in these and other states are available at fractracker. org/map. For more information on special places at risk from gas development, visit outdoors.org/shale.

In response to these and other forces at work against the natural landscape of the Mid-Atlantic, AMC has worked to protect and increase access to wild land in the region. The Highlands Coalition—an alliance of nearly 200 organizations, of which AMC is a leading member—successfully supported the passage of the federal Highlands Conservation Act in 2004, which authorized $100 million in federal matching funds over ten years for land preservation in Pennsylvania, New Jersey, New York, and Connecticut as well as $10 million over 10 years for U.S. Forest Service research and programs. Thanks to this legislation, 3.5 million acres of the Mid-Atlantic Highlands are federally designated for their unique natural and recreational values, with over 4,000 acres having been permanently protected since 2004. AMC works to secure state and federal funding for open space protection—including the viewshed from New York's Bear Mountain (Trip 19)—and suggests to states how and where to fund major trail projects from rural backcountry trails to more urban, multiuse trail systems.

AMC is also collaboratively planning a trail network that will extend from the existing Highlands Trail in New York and New Jersey from the Delaware River at Rieglesville, Pennsylvania, south over 200 miles to the Maryland border. This Pennsylvania Highlands Trail Network will also link existing trails—including Horse-Shoe Trail, the Mason-Dixon Trail system, and the Appalachian Trail—and connect adjacent protected and undisturbed lands throughout the greenway.

For more information on AMC's work in the Mid-Atlantic, visit outdoors. org/conservation/wherewework/highlands/.

SAFETY, GEAR, AND TRIP PLANNING

VENTURING INTO THE WOODS INVOLVES RISK. You need the preparation, fitness, and knowledge to handle those risks. This chapter will prepare you for adventures in the outdoors.

TIPS FOR STAYING SAFE WHILE BACKPACKING

If you follow these simple guidelines, you will be much safer in the outdoors.

Leave an Itinerary. Always tell somebody where you are hiking and when you plan to return. Carry only a photocopied trail description, and leave this book at home; it can give your friends and family the resources they need to act fast and reach proper authorities if you fail to return on time. Be sure to sign in at trail registers wherever possible.

Know Your Limits. Know what you're able to do and where your limits are, no matter how strong a hiker you are. Experience is all about knowing where those limits are, and knowing where you can push and where you shouldn't. Build slowly toward more strenuous trails, and for more challenging hikes, build in extra safety measures, such as bringing a few, more experienced friends along. Ed Viesturs, the first American to summit all fourteen of the world's 8,000-meter peaks, is famous for exercising caution and once turned back just meters away from a summit: "Getting to the summit is optional, but getting back down safely is mandatory." Turning back in the face of weather and physical strain is a mark of an excellent outdoorsperson.

Always Hike with a Buddy. Having a friend along improves your chances of survival if something dangerous happens. If you do end up hiking alone, invest in the added insurance of a rescue beacon. Reassuring "all is well" messages can be emailed to your loved ones or posted directly to Facebook, along with your latitude and longitude. If you ever did need help, a rescue beacon can help ensure that the right people know about it in a flash.

Choose Your Companions Wisely. Hike with people you trust, and try to hike with people who share your inclinations for pace, day length, start time, and more, as you will be more likely to work well as a group. Make sure that each member of the group has a copy of the map and understands the route before you leave the trailhead. Share gear evenly to distribute weight and responsibility.

Stay Together. Even if you and your companions hike at different paces, avoid splitting up. Should something go wrong, communicating up and down the trail can be difficult or impossible, allowing problems to multiply. If essential gear is spread out between slower hikers in need and faster hikers who are farther along the trail, issues could escalate from uncomfortable to serious. At least wait for all members of your group at all trail junctions or places where someone could unknowingly lose track of the trail.

Obsess About the Weather. Study the best weather reports you can get, and plan accordingly. Then plan for it to be a little worse than predicted—it often is.

Know Your Maps; Know Your Trail. Accurate topographic maps and a compass are must-haves for any hiker's gear list. If you're a beginner, familiarize yourself with the skill of following a blazed trail. When you're on-trail, keep your eye out for the blazes. Pay attention to double blazes, as they may indicate turns. If you feel like you haven't seen a blaze in a while, stop and turn around: very often, a blaze for a hiker headed the opposite direction can help guide you. In areas where blazes are few and far between, it can make sense to scout ahead to see if you can pick up a blaze. Always backtrack to the last blaze if you know you've missed the trail; walking in the wrong direction can turn a minor misstep into a search and rescue mission.

Plan for Something to Go Wrong. No matter how well you think you have planned, the wilderness can surprise you. Know how to keep dangerous situations from escalating and how to reach emergency services if they do.

PHYSICAL DANGERS

A backpacking trip is usually not a death-defying experience, but there are some physical dangers you should be aware of and be prepared to counter.

Hypothermia. A life-threatening condition caused by exposure to the wind and the rain, hypothermia is caused when the body's core temperature begins to drop. The symptoms are fatigue, slurred speech, confused thought, and uncontrollable shivering. It doesn't take freezing weather to make conditions dangerous; hikers can become hypothermic in temperatures in the 30s, 40s, and even the 50s with rain and wind.

If you have a choice, don't go out in weather that would put you at risk of hypothermia. If you do choose to hike, make sure your clothing insulates even when wet and that you wearing wind-breaking layers. Keep moving, as vigorous movement can do a great deal to stave off hypothermia. When you camp, get out of the wind quickly, change into your dry things, get warm, and brew hot beverages; do not drink alcohol. Do your best to keep dry throughout your trip.

If you or your partner becomes hypothermic, stop, set up shelter, and get out of wet clothes and into dry ones. Then, get into a sleeping bag, and start brewing hot drinks. Boil water for a bottle and tuck the bottle into the sleeping bag. Eating food will also help raise the body's core temperature.

Heatstroke. The opposite of hypothermia, heatstroke occurs when the body loses control of its ability to regulate its temperature and starts to overheat. Symptoms of heatstroke include cramping, experiencing headaches, or feeling confused.

In the Mid-Atlantic summer, you should take the possibility of heatstroke seriously. Plan to carry extra water, and add electrolytes to your water to help you stay hydrated. Also, wear protective clothing, especially if your trail will be exposed to sun.

If you or your partner does start to suffer from heatstroke, find a way to cool off as soon as possible: either find a creek to soak in, soak the victim's clothes in cool water and fan them, or get the victim into the shade. Provide him or her with cooling drinks until the symptoms subside. In any case, you need to seek medical attention as rapidly as possible.

Water Crossings. Hikers tend to underestimate the potential dangers posed by river and stream crossings. This book notes Mid-Atlantic stream crossings that could become dangerous at certain times of the year, along with descriptions of how to get around such flooded rivers if necessary. Still, considerable rainfall can change any water crossing dramatically. Water flowing above your midthigh has the power to sweep you off your feet; if you are swept away with your clothes and pack on, staying above water can be exhausting if not impossible.

When you make water crossings, take the time to look for the broadest, slowest-moving, shallowest section. Do not cross above a waterfall. When crossing, undo your pack straps so you can get out quickly in case of a fall. Use trekking poles to aid your balance. Accept the fact that you're going to get wet, and take action to mitigate that. Some hikers are trained to remove their shoes, socks, and pants, but crossing some streams barefoot can be equally dangerous. Instead of going barefoot, use special crossing shoes or plan to walk in wet shoes. If getting your trousers wet concerns you, remove them for the crossing.

If you're planning on hiking in a place with serious stream crossings, practice with a partner, as there are techniques that multiple people can use to improve their crossings. You should not have to use such an advanced technique for the trips in this book.

Sunburn. Always wear sunscreen with an SPF of 30 or more. It's also a good idea to wear a sun hat of some sort as well.

PLANT HAZARDS

The Mid-Atlantic has its fair share of plants that want to hurt you. Here are a few of the likely candidates.

Stinging Nettle. During the spring and summer months, you'll need to watch out for this plant. It can grow 1–2 meters tall and is perhaps best identified by its serrated leaves that cause a harmless but unpleasant itching sensation when brushed against skin. Wash with water immediately after being stung. You can avoid being stung by ensuring that your limbs are covered adequately.

Poison Ivy. The urushiol oil in poison ivy poses a serious danger to hikers. The plant grows throughout the Mid-Atlantic, and the rash it causes is long-lasting. Learn to identify this plant to prevent contact. Either a low-lying shrub or a climbing vine, poison ivy has glossy leaves that turn bright red in fall. It also has a hairy vine. (Remember the adage "Hairy vine, no friend of mine!") It grows where it has plenty of sunshine, such as open meadows and broad trail corridors. If you are exposed to poison ivy, wash thoroughly and try to clean your clothes. If you have a severe case, you'll need to see your doctor.

Berries. No matter how inviting those berries dangling over the trail may seem, do not eat them unless you can identify them with full confidence. Mid-Atlantic trails may boast huckleberries and blackberries in season, but nightshade and pokeweed also grow abundantly.

If you'd like to learn more about plants in the region (with pictures to help identify them), the U.S. Department of Agriculture maintains a helpful database at plants.usda.gov/java/. Just search by common or scientific name.

WILDLIFE HAZARDS

Dangerous animal encounters in the Mid-Atlantic are rare, though wildlife is abundant. Nonetheless, there are a few things you need to know about Mid-Atlantic wildlife.

Black Bears. Black bears are rather common in the Mid-Atlantic. Several trips in this book are located in areas with healthy bear populations, and if you hike enough, you're quite likely to see one.

Black bears are, by and large, timid creatures that are definitely not looking for a fight with a human being. If you encounter one on the trail, don't panic or run. Slowly back away; the bear will likely do the same. If a black bear does confront you, make yourself as large as possible (wave your poles!) and slowly back away. Making loud noises can help frighten away the animal. Always avoid a female with cubs.

Never keep food inside your tent. Instead, hang a bear line or use a bear box if you're staying at a shelter that has one. If you are visiting an area with more stringent bear rules, such as the Adirondacks, always follow them. Never feed any wild animal. Habituating a bear, in particular, to human food can lead to dangerous interactions with humans and could eventually get the bear killed.

Ticks. Unfortunately, these little insects present a much more serious danger to hikers than bears. Though several species of ticks live in the Mid-Atlantic, only deer ticks can transmit Lyme disease, a dangerous bacterial infection. This insect is so small that most people who contract Lyme disease never see the tick that bit them. Symptoms of Lyme disease in humans may include fatigue, chills, fever, muscle and joint pain, swollen lymph nodes, and a blotchy skin rash that produces a target-like pattern. If you experience these symptoms, contact your doctor immediately.

To prevent tick bites, first become aware of their habitat and behavior. Ticks love brushy areas, and they latch on to skin and clothing, especially during spring. Wear pants and long-sleeved shirts whenever possible, and treat your clothing with permethrin. If you enjoy cowboy camping or sleeping under a tarp, add a bug bivy to your gear. Always perform tick checks during spring and summer. If you find a tick, do not try to pull it out with your fingers, as you could leave some tick parts under the skin. Instead, using tweezers (part of a first aid kit or on a knife), gently pull out the tick by lifting from the base of the body, where it is attached.

Flies, Gnats, and Mosquitoes. In spring, the Mid-Atlantic can be swarming with all manner of irritating flying insects. They pose no dire threat, but they will drive you crazy. Precautions taken for ticks will keep your body free of bites, but also consider purchasing a head net to keep flying insects away from your face.

Small Mammals. Raccoons, skunks, porcupines, foxes, and mice pose no danger to hikers, but they will go after your food, sometimes gnawing through an expensive piece of gear to get it. To prevent this sort of damage, hang your food on a bear line, use a food locker or a bear canister, or use a mouse-proof line at a shelter.

Giardia. If you drink contaminated water or exercise poor backcountry hygiene, you could develop a nasty gastro-intestinal problem caused by the bacteria *Giardia lamblia.* Symptoms include diarrhea, flatulence, foul-smelling excrement, nausea, fatigue, and abdominal cramps. Treat water on the trail, especially from sources near shelters, camping areas, and other heavily used locations. Use hand sanitizer to ensure that you don't cross contaminate your food, water, or gear.

GEAR: EQUIPPING YOURSELF FOR THE BACKCOUNTRY

For better or worse, backpacking is an activity where the gear matters, and some money must be spent before you can head out into the woods. What matters even more is your skill with your equipment. Some backpackers spend a few thousand dollars on rarely used gear that would really be suitable for the high Himalaya or the Arctic; others rack up night after night in the backcountry with well-worn gear. Make no mistake: you'd rather be the person with the battered but well-loved gear.

The subject of backcountry equipment could fill its own book. This section is simply a primer that will introduce beginners to the basics and possibly save more experienced hikers time and money.

A few quick disclaimers. First, this discussion of gear is oriented to three-season (spring, summer, and fall) use in the states discussed in this book: New York, Pennsylvania, Delaware, New Jersey, Maryland, Virginia, and West Virginia. Winter backpacking is a great adventure, but there are specialized considerations and equipment for those trips that are not covered here. See *AMC's Guide to Winter Hiking and Camping* if you want to expand your trips into the fourth season.

Second, this primer leans toward ultra-light, or minimalist, equipment. I do believe that the lighter your load, the happier you are likely to be on the trail, but only you are responsible for taking the equipment appropriate to the environment and weather you're likely to face. Your safety (and comfort) is far more important than meeting anyone's expectations about how much you should carry. With that said, new backpackers often carry extra weight that does not meaningfully contribute to their safety and that may, in some cases, even compromise it. Too often, beginner backpackers purchase heavy, unnecessary equipment, find themselves miserable carrying it, and let their equipment limit their view of their ability on the trail. Certainly, heavier is not better.

A useful way to think of your gear is to divide it into systems that perform necessary functions on the trail. The functions are shelter, sleep, carry, cook, hygiene, clothing, and other gear essentials.

Shelter

The most common shelter choice for backpackers in the Mid-Atlantic is a three-season tent consisting of a waterproof outer fly, an interior made largely of mesh, a collapsible pole skeleton, and stakes to anchor it to the ground. High-quality, lightweight tents for one or two people can weigh as little as 2–3 pounds. Usually, the less you spend, the more the tent will weigh, so buy the lightest shelter you can afford. A good three-season tent of this type can be an effective and trustworthy companion through many, many trips. Treat it as an investment and you'll reap the dividends.

Buying a tent with all the bells and whistles often means that you're buying a heavy tent, but there are some features you should consider. Check to see that the tent you're considering has some vestibule room (essentially space between the fly and the tent) in which you can store boots and other gear. If the seams of your tent do not come factory sealed, seal them yourself. If the manufacturer of your tent offers a ground sheet that is pre-cut for the tent, purchasing it can be a wise decision.

Learn how to pitch your tent before you venture into the woods. Most are fairly intuitive, but even advanced backpackers can be flummoxed by a new pitching arrangement. You don't want to set it up for the first time alone on a dark, cold, wet backcountry night.

Shelters cut for just one person are fine, but two-person versions offer extra space to stash equipment, a friend, or a canine companion for just a few more ounces of weight. As backpacking tents are small, a few extra inches between yourself and the walls of the tent can help on a night when you're having issues with condensation.

More adventuresome hikers might consider more minimalist shelters such as tarps, hammocks, and bivy sacks. These types of lightweight options each have their own advantages and disadvantages. Often used by climbers, bivvies are waterproof sacks that can be placed around a sleeping bag; though they are constrictive, they are very light and can get the job done. A hammock combines a shelter and a sleep system that hangs between two trees. Some vastly prefer the quality of sleep they get in a hammock and, of course, you never have to worry about rocky or uneven tent sites. There is no shortage of trees in the Mid-Atlantic! Tarps can serve as very lightweight shelters that are not fully enclosed; in the Mid-Atlantic, they can be enough for nine or ten months out of the year. If one of these alternative shelters sounds appealing to you, do some research and test one out on a mild night. They are not for everybody, but many backpackers swear by them.

Sleep

Most backpackers carry a sleeping bag and pad combination. Both are necessary pieces of equipment that are designed to work together. The pad is designed to insulate the bag from the cold ground, not primarily for comfort. Novice backpackers sometimes confuse the pad for a luxury item and think they can save weight by leaving it out. Even in August, this is a miserable way to spend the night; in November, you're likely to be up all night tending the fire. No one ever makes this mistake twice.

When it comes to sleeping pads, you have a lot of options, including some that can save you money. Foam pads are cheap, virtually indestructible, and adequate for getting the job done. Many new inflatable pads are warm, lightweight, and almost ridiculously comfortable. Unfortunately, they are more expensive and they can be punctured. If you find yourself on the fence on this topic, just buy a foam pad and see how it works—they are so cheap there's no risk.

Before you purchase, evaluate a pad's R-value, which estimates how well the pad insulates you from the cold ground. An R-value from 2.8 to 3.4 is fine for three-season use in the Mid-Atlantic. You can also choose to buy pads that cover half, three-quarters, or all of your body.

Sleeping bags also offer choices that affect the price you'll pay. First, decide whether you'll purchase a goose down–insulated sleeping bag or one insulated with synthetic material. Down bags are warm for their weight, highly compressible, and have great longevity. They are also quite expensive, and if they become wet, they lose their ability to insulate. Synthetic bags are much cheaper and continue to insulate when wet, but they do not compress well and are slightly heavier for their warmth. Ultimately, this choice may come down to how often you intend to use your bag. A down bag is a great investment for enthusiastic hikers. If you're only planning to backpack a few nights a year, it might make more sense to save the money and buy a synthetic bag. Also look for bags that have a durable water resistant (DWR) finish to them. You may not have much trouble keeping your down bag dry, but a little extra insurance never hurt. Some environments are just wet (Pennsylvania, I'm looking at you!), and you'll often have condensation to deal with. A stronger finish on a down bag is well worth the cash.

For three-season use in the Mid-Atlantic (and, indeed, for many other purposes), if you're going to own only one bag, buy a 20-degree bag. The bag will be comfortable in spring and fall, and it will give you insurance in the shoulder season if temperatures unexpectedly drop below freezing. It will be too warm in summer, but you can just drape it over you like a blanket. Of course, take your own hiking habits and comfort into consideration. If you know you'll never be outdoors if there's a chance of a freeze, then you might just get a 35-degree bag. If you know you are often cold, you might need a 15- or even a 10-degree bag.

Try to evaluate a bag using its European Norm (EN) 13537 testing rating. Many U.S. retailers are switching to this system because it provides much more useful and objective information about how a bag will perform for men and women at different temperatures. The EN 13537 system tries to objectively answer questions about differences in how a man or a woman will experience sleeping in the bag at different temperatures, eliminating some of the guesswork of evaluating bags based on the (manufacturer's) temperature rating alone.

Remember that you can supplement the insulation of any sleeping bag by wearing additional clothes or by adding a liner. So, if you buy a 35-degree bag and decide that you do want to do a November trip, no worries. Just pack a few extra layers.

Carry
Logically, this section puts the "backpack" in "backpacking." Traditional wisdom for new backpackers recommends a backpack with 3,500 to 4,000 cubic inches of capacity. Following this advice at a major outdoors store will lead you to an internal frame pack with an assortment of features—pockets, hydration sleeves, exterior loops, sleeping bag compartments, and so on. Some of these features may be useful, but many of them won't be. They all add weight. It is perfectly possible to buy a pack that weighs 5–7 pounds, all by itself.

For a lighter approach, a 3,000-cubic-inch (or 50-liter) pack for a trip of three days and two nights should be about right. A simple sack on a simple frame can be enough for a weekend trip. If you decide to pursue longer, more aggressive trips later, you are likely to need another, larger pack beyond a small, minimalist one, but you'll appreciate having a lighter option as you gain skill, stamina, and experience. Most of the trips in this book can be completed with a small weekend pack, and all of them are possible if you're willing to section-hike some of the longer ones. With some experience under your belt, you'll eventually find it easy to pack for a three-to-five-day trip even in a weekend pack.

When you're trying on any pack, ensure that it fits you properly and that you try it with weight in the pack. Choosing the correct size is tricky because it relies on your torso length, which, unlike your inseam, is not a measurement you're used to giving. In stores, a good salesperson will measure your torso and will fill an appropriately sized pack with weight.

When first putting on the pack, loosen the shoulder straps, and then position the hip belt so that it sits on the top of your hips. Tighten the hip belt so that all the weight is on your hips. The shoulder straps should rise up above your shoulders before coming down behind them. Snug up the shoulder straps, tighten the load lifter straps (which pull the top of the pack toward you), and attach and tighten the sternum strap. Then take a walk around the store to see how it feels. Almost no weight should be resting on your shoulders. The weight should instead be resting on your hips, as your legs are far stronger and able to carry the load far easier. Remember that a small, niggling issue—even a little chafing or neck pain—is likely to be really quite catastrophic after ten miles uphill, with a heavy load, over slippery rocks.

When you purchase your pack, consider your options for weatherproofing it. Though a store-bought pack cover is one route, the easiest, simplest, cheapest, lightest, and most effective way to keep your gear dry is to use large trash compactor or contractor bags from a hardware store as a pack liner. Not only are these bags cheap, but they also work much better than a pack cover, which may only cover part of the pack. If inclement weather is in the forecast, consider bringing an extra dry sack for your sleeping bag and sleeping clothes.

When you load your pack at home, keep the heaviest items toward the back of the pack and lower down, as close to your center of gravity as possible. As you pack, the lighter items should be placed higher and farther to the front of the pack. Of course, such a packing scheme must be balanced by your need to get to items you'll need. There is some art to it all. As you get more practice with your pack, you'll get better at it.

In the "old days," when external frame packs were far more common, your tent (or shelter of choice) could be strapped onto the outside of your pack, allowing you to quickly set up camp in the worst weather without ever exposing the inside of the pack. You probably won't be using an external frame pack, but try to stow your shelter where you can get to it and pitch it easily.

Cook

Hikers' diverse attitudes about backcountry comfort manifest most obviously in their attitudes toward food. Some want to cook elaborate meals on an open fire; others expect stove-cooked pancakes; and a hardy few will go stoveless and survive entirely on a diet of ramen and chocolate bars. As always, hike your own hike: the following advice is just one of many options you have.

Kitchen Gear. If you'd rather be walking than camping and are happy to be the earliest starter on the trail, opt for a quick, easy cook system that relies simply on boiling water. Boil-a-bag meals can be quite toothsome, and with the addition of some dry soups, instant coffee, and some powdered hot drinks, you can start and end your days with warm food and a full stomach.

Self-contained, all-in-one stoves that sit on isobutane-propane canisters work well for light packers on weekend trips. The best kind have an integrated cup that also serves as a pot; there are a few competing brands. Such stoves are light, fairly cheap, safe, reliable, and easy to use. They also boil quickly, and a single canister is more than adequate to supply hot water for two on a weekend trip.

If you're not a fan of fuel canisters (it can be tough to determine how much fuel is left in one of them, so you end up carrying too much), try an alcohol stove. Search online for "alcohol stove" or check out thesodacanstove.com. You could make your own, or you could order some very nice, yet inexpensive, models online. These stoves are about the lightest possible, very cheap, quite reliable, and boil water quickly. Best of all, you can fill a small plastic bottle with fuel from a much larger container that you leave at home. You can also buy fuel for them at gas stations around the world.

Dishes and cutlery for these types of systems can be minimal. All-in-one stoves often come with food-grade cups for hot drinks and oatmeal, and boiled meals can be eaten out of the bags they come in. A plastic or titanium spork is enough for most meals. This approach produces little trash and few dishes to clean.

Food. Carrying about 1.5–2 pounds of food per person per day will sustain hikers through even very vigorous days without adding too much additional weight. Dehydrated dinners make meal planning relatively easy. Choose the ones you like, add your preferred breakfast drinks and food, and choose daytime foods that can be eaten while walking without any preparation, like granola, Gorp, chocolate, sports beans, and jerky. Don't deny yourself a luxury item like powdered cider, coffee, an avocado, or dried cherries, and make sure that you take only food you heartily enjoy. Dial in your food rationing for your own appetite and needs. It takes some practice, so keep careful track of how much food goes uneaten on your trips.

Do invest in a lightweight stuff sack to use as a food bag. Add line to the sack to hang it away from bears' reach or use it to keep your food together and easy to find in a shelter's bear box.

Water Carrying Capacity. With the exception of a few ridges (which are well noted in this book), the Mid-Atlantic offers backpackers an abundance of water sources. Usually, you'll need a carrying capacity of just 2–3 liters (having the third is nice if you plan to camp at a dry spot), but you'll rarely need to carry more than 2. While it's very important to stay well hydrated, carrying more water than you need only adds extra weight.

Save your money: do not buy heavy, thick, rigid plastic water bottles. If you are determined to spend the money, *soft* plastic bottles fold up and are much lighter. Honestly, though, plastic bottles from the recycling bin work just fine. Do be aware, when you're choosing your system, that it's sometimes nice to have a wide mouth on a bottle, and some water treatment methods more or less require it.

Many hikers, backpackers, and other outdoors types of various stripes eschew bottles for bladder systems. A soft plastic bladder of water sits in a sleeve in your pack; a tube extends out of the bladder and reaches in front of the pack, allowing you to sip as you desire. You are more likely to drink more with the easy access of a bladder, so you're likely to stay well hydrated. On the other hand, you'll find it hard to ration correctly because the bladder is hidden in your pack, and you may be surprised by how much (or little!) water you've consumed at the end of a day.

Water Treatment. Always treat the water you take from backcountry sources. Luckily and unluckily, the many treatment options available to you have pros and cons, including:

- Pump filters (good for a large group, but heavy and prone to cracking in winter)
- Ultraviolet (UV) lights (light, but finicky and reliant on batteries)
- Gravity-fed filters (gaining in popularity, but slow sometimes)
- Chemical-based systems based on iodine, chlorine, or bleach (simple and cheap, but can affect the water's taste)

Do some thinking about how your treatment system will work with your water containers. If you're using a UV light, a 3-liter bladder won't work by itself, as the light is designed to treat 1 liter at a time. You'll need to add a 1-liter wide-mouth bottle to treat in, and then pour the treated water into the bladder, repeating until the bladder is full.

Hygiene

Though you'll want to be hygienic on your trip, there's no doubt that you're going to get dirtier and smellier than you're used to being in your daily life. It's

OK. A little dirt won't hurt you, and you're likely to feel more comfortable in your skin (however dirty it is) as you gain experience.

You can still address comfort and sanitation on the trail, however. Fill a pint-sized plastic bag with the smallest bottles of the various hygiene-related products you think you absolutely need. The key is repackaging: reuse sample-size shampoo bottles from hotels and try to bring only what you need for the few days you'll be out. You may want to consider bringing any or all of these items:

- Hand sanitizer
- Toothpaste (you can dehydrate blobs of it for an ultra-light solution)
- Floss
- A toothbrush (cut off the handle to reduce weight)
- A little biodegradable soap
- A little biodegradable mouthwash
- Sunscreen
- Anti-chaffing lotion
- Insect repellent (along with a head net, this can be a vital piece of gear in certain situations)
- Any individual prescription medication you really need
- Contact solution, a contact case, and an extra set of contacts
- A bag of toilet paper and doubled bag for dirty toilet paper
- Alcohol-based wet wipes

The prospect of going to the bathroom in the woods causes some people a lot of anxiety. You do get used to it. Always do your business in a six-inch cat hole at least 200 feet from camp, trails, and water sources. No need to carry a trowel for this purpose. A tent stake or a trekking pole works fine. Remember: never discard or bury toilet paper, even the biodegradable kind. While fecal material decays very quickly, toilet paper does not, and it costs you nothing to carry the dirty paper out in a double bag. Nothing is worse than encountering an over-used campsite where the toilet paper is "blooming" from shallow cat holes. In some very high-use areas, you may be required to carry your own fecal waste from campsites. I don't know of any such area in the Mid-Atlantic, however. Do your part to keep campsites clean so we can avoid this sort of regulation.

Clothing

To avoid bringing too much clothing, never carry multiples. Your clothes will be dirty, but that's temporary. Another tactic to keep your pack light is to think of your clothes in two categories: the clothes you wear while walking (that could get wet) and the clothes you wear while in camp (that must stay dry).

Each time you camp, you get out of the walking clothes and switch into the dry clothes.

The fabric of the clothes you bring will matter greatly on the trail, as the wrong choices invite trouble and the right ones help ensure a safe, comfortable trip. Consider the following when you're packing:

- Cotton is a *terrible* fabric for outdoor purposes. It will get wet, either from precipitation, condensation, or perspiration, and when it does, it loses all insulating properties. Even worse, once it's wet, it tends to stay wet. These characteristics account for the deaths by hypothermia of a number of hikers every year. Leave your cotton garments at home.
- Wool fares much better among natural fibers. It continues to insulate when wet, but it does tend to retain quite a lot of water, which makes it heavy. Merino wool is especially valuable as a base layer.
- Nylon and polyester clothing are great choices for outdoor clothing. They dry quickly, wick moisture away from the body, and continue to insulate when wet. Virtually every conceivable manufacturer makes clothing of this sort that is quite suitable.
- Down is wonderful from a warmth-to-weight ratio perspective, but if you get it wet, it is useless. Synthetic puffy thermal layers are available, and recently some manufacturers have begun marketing down that is water repellent.
- Fleece takes a bit of a knock for being heavier than puffy down and synthetic layers, but it insulates well, even when wet, and holds up quite well. Fleece is a vital fabric for outdoor purposes.

On Your Person. Be bold, start cold. You need to be wearing clothes that will leave you a little chilly if you're not moving. Layer your clothes so that you minimize perspiration and yet have the weather protection you need. Admittedly, layering correctly is a bit of an art, and it's an individual thing too, so you'll get better at it with practice.

Here are some of the likely items you'll be wearing at the trailhead:

- Polyester sports underwear
- Nylon hiking trousers, shorts, skirt, or kilt (long pants will protect against insects and plants in the Mid-Atlantic, but shorter garments are better suited for hot days)
- Lightweight synthetic or merino wool base-layer T-shirt
- Lightweight synthetic long-sleeve shirt
- Baseball cap or other sun hat
- Digital sports watch

- Trekking poles (incredibly helpful for crossing rugged ground, descending, climbing, or crossing a stream)

In Your Pack. For three-season purposes, especially when there's little chance of the temperature dipping below freezing, you won't need to carry much in the way of extra clothing. Some of the extra items you should consider include:

- A thermal layer, such as a fleece or down jacket (easily accessible to stay warm when you stop to rest)
- Gloves (fleece gloves work well in mild weather)
- A warm hat
- An extra pair of socks
- A rain jacket and a pair of rain pants (lightweight rain gear is fine for most weather, but for rain when it's in the 30s and 40s, hardshell gear will be more useful)
- A dry base layer, top and bottoms

Except for the rain jacket and pants, these items should be in your weatherproofed pack. Keep the rain jacket and pants where they are easily accessible.

To evaluate your choices, consider the worst weather you could withstand if you put on every stitch of the clothing in your pack. Or imagine perfect hypothermia weather—wind and rain with temperatures in the 30s or 40s—and consider how your gear would withstand it.

On Your Feet. Traditionally, backpackers have been advised to wear large, heavy, waterproof, leather hiking boots. Recent trends have tended to emphasize lightweight footwear, such as trail runners, which are suitable for a fit person with a moderate pack weight through most of the year in the Mid-Atlantic.

The most important thing, however, is that your footwear fit *you* well. Go to the store and try on a lot of different shoes and boots. Walk around in them, and buy the pair that feels the best on your feet. Fit trumps every other consideration.

When buying your shoes or boots, consider your sock situation. If you plan to wear multiple pairs of socks (like a silk or nylon base layer followed by a heavier wool sock, which can limit blistering and improve insulation), you'll need to size the footwear accordingly.

Other Gear Essentials

Up to this point, we've been discussing the big systems that characterize backpacking. Now we're going to dial in on the small stuff, including the must-have essentials for every trip. Keep these items together in a little stuff sack so they can be easily located and moved between packs for your different activities.

Map and Compass. You need the best available map for each trip (listed in each trip description), as well as a compass. Bring several maps if you can, as different maps show different details. A compass is a valuable tool, even if you just use it to make sure you're facing the right way, but your backcountry skills will increase a great deal if you find the time to take a map and compass course. A GPS unit can supplement, but not supplant, these tools and skills.

Illumination. The backpacker's common choice for a light source these days is a headlamp, which leaves your hands free for other purposes. For short trips, you can probably get away without carrying an extra set of batteries, but if you're planning to walk at night, the extra batteries are a must.

Fire. Carrying a few options for emergency fire starting ensures that you can have a heat source in almost any conditions. Consider a cheap lighter, a few waterproof matches, and a firestarter—all protected by plastic bags.

Knife. A small, simple knife with a pair of scissors will be enough for almost every trip in this book.

First Aid Kit. The little premade kits are a good place to start, but you'll want to personalize your kit as your backcountry experience grows. Keep it stocked with plenty of medical tape, ibuprofen, and tough, water-resistant adhesive bandages.

Repair Kit. The backcountry can be tough on gear, so you need to have a few items to conduct emergency field repair on vital equipment. Some extra lengths of guy line, duct tape, a needle, and tough thread can be quite useful. If you carry an inflatable mattress, toss the repair kit that came with it into the bag.

Electronics in the Backcountry

Though they may seem to provide a less rugged experience, electronic devices can actually give hikers a lot of power in the backcountry, enabling better navigation, communication, and documentation. Here is a list of the electronics that are valuable even to lightweight backpackers.

- A camera, whether you prefer a weatherproof point-and-shoot camera or a full-fledged DSLR.
- A handheld GPS unit, which is extremely powerful for both navigation and for documenting your route (but does not replace a map and compass).

- A rescue beacon. A number of recent units allow you to communicate, even when there's not an emergency, so this device really gives your loved ones peace of mind.
- A smartphone, mostly for communication. Several of the smartphones are maturing into fairly good backcountry navigation tools.
- An e-reader. If you suspect you're going to be spending a lot of time in your sleeping bag or at camp, it's nice to have.

With all these devices, units that have long battery life and are waterproof are your best choices. The aggressive application of plastic bags can make the difference for electronic gear not designed for the outdoors.

Base Weight versus Total Weight

Comparing the weight of your gear with other hikers' and between trips can be tough without a firm baseline, so backpackers speak in terms of base weight and total weight. Total weight is the weight of all the equipment you carry on your back as you leave your vehicle and walk into the woods (including consumables like water, food, and fuel). Base weight is the sum total of all the equipment that you always take, minus the consumables. It includes the water bottle, but not the water itself. Base weight is a particularly useful measurement because you can compare the weight of your gear across trips and seasons. By measuring, recording, and comparing your base weight, you can trim unnecessary weight while gearing yourself efficiently for conditions in the Mid-Atlantic.

Hike Light but Hike Smart

An experienced outdoorsperson must always take the pieces of gear that are appropriate for the environment. Those new to the outdoors must temper their desire to carry as little as possible with the recognition that it is better to be safe than sorry. If and when you are ready to drop your pack's weight, the real payoff is reaching a point where your pack weight hardly affects you. Still, the tiers are admittedly arbitrary. A base weight of less than 20 pounds earns you the title of lightweight backpacker, but you can still choose to go lighter. A base weight of less than 10 pounds will qualify you as an ultra-light backpacker; a base weight of less than 5 pounds makes you a super-ultra-light backpacker.

A quick cautionary note: it is possible to take the goal of ultimate lightness too far. If you go into the woods often enough with lightweight gear, you will eventually be carrying a piece of gear too light to get a particular job done, and you'll certainly wish you had decided to bring the more substantial piece of gear.

Don't end up bringing a trash bag for rain gear rather than a hardshell; don't opt for too little water or too little food. Lightweight backpackers call those kinds of decisions "stupid light." See also Andrew Skurka's blog post, "'Stupid light': Why light is not necessarily right, and why lighter is not necessarily better," for a more detailed discussion of these types of errors (andrewskurka. com/2012/stupid-light-not-always-right-or-better).

Packing Checklist
Remember these tips if you choose to lighten your load:
- Know how much your stuff weighs. Invest in a postal scale and weigh each and every item before it goes in your pack.
- Use a permanent marker to write the weight of things on your gear.
- Repeat, mantra-like, "This plastic spork weighs 1.1 ounces, and it is an essential piece of gear."
- Maintain a spreadsheet where you total your base weight. Maintain slightly different spreadsheets for, say, a summer load versus a fall load.
- Keep notes on your spreadsheets about how individual pieces of gear perform. If you find yourself writing "did not use" next to a piece of equipment time and time again, you should reconsider taking it along.
- Read a book. Max Clelland's *Ultralight Backpackin' Tips: 153 Amazing & Inexpensive Tips for Extremely Lightweight Camping* is one of several respected options. That book will cover lightweight backpacking far more thoroughly than this primer.

LEAVE NO TRACE

It's vital that we, as good outdoorspeople, take care of our forests and mountains for future generations. Follow these simple guidelines to "leave no trace" of your passage:

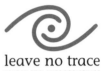

- **Do Not Scar the Land.** Do not cut switchbacks. Stay on the trail. Leave rocks, plants, and other natural objects as you find them. If you do end up off-trail, spread out to minimize the environmental damage of your passage.
- **Camping.** Camp only at established sites. Do not dig ditches around your tent. Keep your camp clean and never leave food out. Contain activities to where there is no vegetation. When you strike camp, try to return the natural environment to the way you found it.
- **Fires.** Campfires, when allowed, should always be made in an established fire ring. You should never create a new fire ring. Collect only dead or downed wood. Make sure the fire is completely out before leaving.
- **Sanitation.** When defecating, choose a spot at least 200 feet from trails, water sources, and campsites. Dig a cat hole six inches deep, do your business, and cover it with the soil you removed. Do not bury toilet paper; carry it out with you.
- **Washing.** To wash yourself or your dishes, carry water 200 feet away from streams or lakes. Scatter strained dishwater. Avoid the use of soap, if possible; otherwise use only small amounts of biodegradable soap. At all costs, keep soap out of creeks and streams.
- **Garbage.** Carry out all garbage and burn only paper. Thoroughly inspect your site for trash and spilled food before leaving.
- **Group Size.** Keep groups small to minimize impact.
- **Animals.** Do not feed wildlife. Observe only from a distance.

- **Noise.** Be respectful of others in the wilderness. Listen to the sounds of nature.

For those interested in learning more, AMC provides training in Leave No Trace ethics. Visit outdoors.org/recreation/leadership/lnt.

1

VIRGINIA

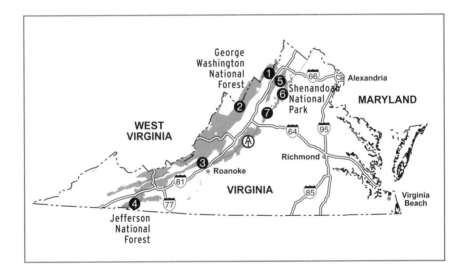

TRIP 1
BIRD'S EYE VIEW

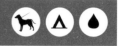

Location: George Washington and Jefferson National Forests, Virginia
Highlights: Ridge walking to Tibbet Knob and a high campsite with a panoramic view of the Alleghenies
Distance: 3.1 miles round-trip
Total Elevation Gain/Loss: 1,001 feet gain/1,001 feet loss
Trip Length: 2 days
Difficulty: Moderate with two short stretches of scrambling
Recommended Maps:
- National Geographic, *Trails Illustrated Map for Massanutten and Great North Mountain*, 792.
- Potomac Appalachian Trail Club, *Map F. Trails in Great North Mountain—North Half of George Washington National Forest*, 6th ed. Vienna, VA: Potomac Appalachian Trail Club, 2004.
- Potomac Appalachian Trail Club, *Guide to Great North Mountain Trails*, 2nd ed. Ed. Glenn Palatini and Wil Kohlbrenner. Vienna, VA: Potomac Appalachian Trail Club, 2008.
- USGS Quad: Wolf Gap.

Enjoy a quick jaunt walking along the ridge that defines the border between Virginia and West Virginia. Less frequently visited than neighboring Big Schloss, the views of the Alleghenies from Tibbet Knob are second to none.

HIKE OVERVIEW
The out-and-back walk to Tibbet Knob is an excellent excursion for a beginner backpacker, a more veteran backpacker with limited time, or someone just wanting to shake out a new piece of gear in the field. Not only is the view from the knob quite fine—one of the best in the region, really—but also the walking is fairly easy. Beginners will find the two short sections of scrambling a worthy challenge. To cap it off, an excellent backcountry campsite is located at the knob itself. Pitch a tent and dine while enjoying a sunset view. Given its brevity, this would be a good hike to carry along some more toothsome (and weighty) food. Since there's no water anywhere along the ridge, you'll have to carry in your water. Individual water needs vary, but I'd recommend 3 liters each for the short hike in, dinner, breakfast, and the short hike out.

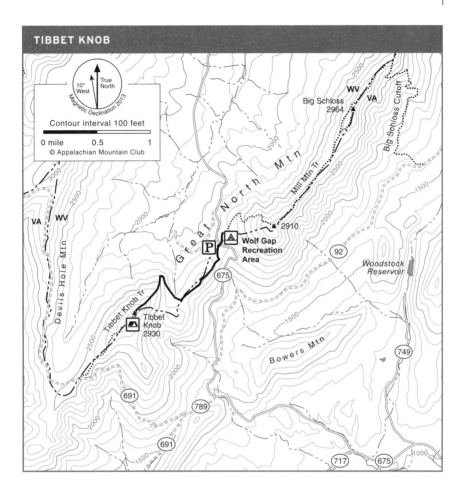

OVERNIGHT OPTIONS

Backcountry camping is allowed throughout George Washington National Forest. Never create a new fire ring, and always follow Forest Service rules and Leave No Trace procedures. There is no need for a camping permit, but keep your group size relatively small.

Tibbet Knob Backcountry Site (1.71/2,930/38° 54.922' N, 78° 42.276' W). Standing on top of Tibbet Knob and eying the westward view, turn left and continue south on the orange-blazed trail just a few feet. The campsite is on the left. This attractive spot is centered around a fire ring, but it is rather narrow—it will accommodate two 2–3 person backpacking tents, but anything more will be a squeeze.

Wolf Gap Campground (0.0/2,240/38° 55.469' N, 78° 41.343' W). As Wolf Gap Road passes over the Virginia–West Virginia border, you'll see a sign for the Wolf Gap Recreation Area. The nine pleasant sites are free, but they go quickly on a pretty autumn day; if you plan to camp here, try to arrive earlier rather than later. Each site has a parking spot, tent pad, picnic table, and fire ring. There is a privy. Day-hikers make their way through the campsite in order to hike to Big Schloss.

HOW TO REACH THE TRAILHEAD

Driving south on I-81, take Exit 283 in Woodstock, Virginia, and head west on VA 42 for about 5 miles. Turn right onto Union Church Road, and then continue (left) on Back Road/VA 623. Turn right onto VA 675 (Wolf Gap Road), and drive about 6 miles to Wolf Gap Recreation Area. Turn into the day-hikers' parking lot on the right and park (38° 55.4482' N, 78° 41.3572' W).

HIKE DESCRIPTION

From the parking lot, you have the option of walking through the campsite, which takes you to the trail for Big Schloss, or crossing VA 675. Cross the road. You'll see a sign for Tibbet Knob. The orange-blazed trail passes a primitive campsite on the right, but it's too close to the road to be ideal. Very soon (about 0.2 mi), the trail begins a steady but not steep climb. You've reached the top of this climb when you have your first view of the Massanutten and Blue Ridge mountains on your left (0.5/2,439). At this point you'll be walking a fairly typical Virginia ridge. Looking ahead you can see a knob that the trail will round on the right before climbing Tibbet Knob itself.

The trail descends briefly and shortly, and then evens out. Like many of the mountains in this area (Massanutten Mountain come to mind), the footing is rather rocky, so take care. As the trail winds around the knob, it passes through a forested area. Eventually, the trail will begin to climb a bit, and you'll have obscured views to the left and the right. After a switchback, it climbs more aggressively to the ridgeline.

About a quarter-mile from the summit of Tibbet Knob (1.3/2,754), a quick turn in the trail will take you to the first stretch of rocky scrambles. While scrambling can be dangerous, these areas are not especially worrisome. On the descent, they may require more caution. The first scramble is no more than 50 or 60 feet long and is followed by relatively even ground. The second, steeper scramble comes very near the summit (1.5/2,866).

Pass through some thick woods, and then emerge on top of Tibbet Knob (1.6/2,930/38° 54.8560' N, 78° 42.2994' W). The rocky outcropping enjoys a beautiful 180-degree view to the west, including Big Schloss in the north and Devil's Hole Mountain in the northwest. The campsite is just past the summit. The next morning, simply return the way you came.

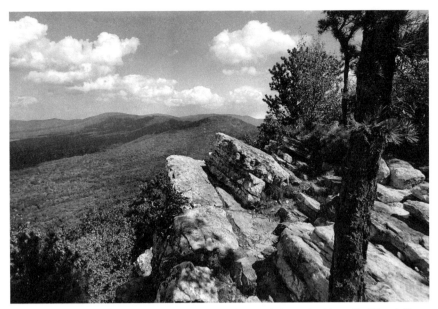

Tibbet Knob's summit provides a splendid vantage point overlooking all of Trout Run Valley.

OTHER OPTIONS

If you enjoyed the little scrambles needed to reach Tibbet Knob, do some additional scrambling from your campsite. A few rocky outcroppings that look easterly and produce an almost-360-degree view can be reached from just below the second scramble. These are considerably more difficult than the scrambles on the trail, so leave your pack and use caution.

Adding another night out is relatively easy in this area. After spending the night at Tibbet Knob, return to Wolf Gap, pitch your tent again in one of the free campsites, and then do the hike to Big Schloss. This 4-mile hike also features some nice views. Alternatively, camp out beyond Big Schloss. For the truly adventuresome, there is a campsite on top of Big Schloss itself.

NEARBY

I-81 in Woodstock, Virginia, has the usual array of big box retail stores and chain restaurants, but there are also plenty of options for local fare.

ADDITIONAL INFORMATION

U.S. Forest Service; North River Ranger District; 401 Oakwood Drive; Harrisonburg, VA 22801-9999; 540-432-0187

TRIP 2
AMPHIBIOUS LANDING

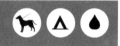

Location: Ramseys Draft Wilderness, George Washington and Jefferson National Forests, Virginia

Highlights: Old growth forest in the Wilderness, splashing through crossings of Ramseys Draft and the North River, ridgeline views of the Appalachian highlands

Distance: 44 miles round-trip

Total Elevation Gain/Loss: 10,461 feet gain/10,461 feet loss

Trip Length: 3–6 days

Difficulty: Challenging

Recommended Maps and Other Resources:

- National Geographic, Trails Illustrated Map for Massanutten and Great North Mountain, 792.
- USGS Quads: West Augusta, Stokesville, Palo Alto, and Reddish Knob.

Along the border between Virginia and West Virginia, the knobs stand higher, the drafts run swifter, and the forests grow wilder than farther east. This walk weaves together ridgelines, distant vistas, and river gorges with abundant stream crossings. In the upper reaches of Ramseys Draft—a federally designated Wilderness area—backpackers will visit one of the last remaining stands of old-growth giant hemlocks on the East Coast.

HIKE OVERVIEW

By linking together the trails in the Ramseys Draft Wilderness with 26.2-mile Wild Oak National Recreation Trail, this route creates a sustained journey in the high country of Central Virginia. Together, the trails form a lopsided figure-eight centered on the beautiful camping at Hiner Spring. You'll begin by climbing the wet and wonderful Ramseys Draft with its innumerable crossings. From there, follow Wild Oak Trail as it heads counterclockwise to reach far-ranging, mountainous vistas and the cooling waters of the North River. Upon your return to Hiner Spring, you descend to the trailhead via gentle Shenandoah Mountain Trail, with more views of the draft's drainage and the Alleghenies in the west.

If valley of Ramseys Draft, with its maze of unmarked trails, gigantic deadfalls, and endless stream crossings, seems excessively wild, keep in mind that the trail's primitive condition is a direct result of Wilderness designation, where you will find fewer blazes, signs, and bridges than you would find on other trails. You may very well wonder about the wisdom of that particular decision as you ford the twenty-odd stream crossings. Be prepared for these crossings; in some seasons, even the most skilled rockhoppers will get wet.

Ramseys Draft does have something of a Jekyll-and-Hyde temperament. If you time your visit well, a late spring visit should mean there's plenty of water, but not so much that crossings are as dangerous as they can be earlier in spring. At this prime time of year, the vegetation hasn't yet grown thick enough to begin choking out the trail. Much of your experience may depend on what recent maintenance has been done and if the blowdowns have been cleared. If not, you'll wish you had a machete, or a chainsaw.

Despite the trail's wildness and the absence of blazes in the Wilderness, you should have no trouble finding your way. The steep sides of the gorge mean that you have only to continue walking in the gully to make headway. Cairns do mark some of the more confusing points, and trail junctions are signed.

HOW TO REACH THE TRAILHEAD

After heading south on I-81, take Exit 225 and turn right onto VA 262/ Woodrow Wilson Parkway, which will allow you to bypass Staunton. Just west of town, bear right onto US 250. About 20 miles farther west, you'll spot a trailhead for Ramseys Draft. Turn into the picnic ground, but drive straight past the day use area to the gravel parking lot beyond (38° 18.482' N, 79° 21.673' W).

OVERNIGHT OPTIONS

Alongside the plentiful opportunities for primitive camping (no permits required), the area features several developed campsites suitable for vehicle camping. Additionally, you will see many unofficial campsites, of varying quality, along SR 715 and Forest Road 95.

Ramseys Draft (1.2/2,385/38° 19.160' N, 79° 20.932' W). Ramseys Draft Trail offers no shortage of attractive camping sites, which will be especially tempting if you're arriving late. Several are just a few hundred yards from the trailhead.

Hiner Spring (6.2/3,986/38° 22.277' N, 79° 19.056' W). In the meadow where rivulets converge to form the draft, you'll find an excellent backcountry camping spot with many tent sites and a built-up fire pit. Walk a few hundred feet up the back of the meadow toward Hardscrabble Knob for an especially beautiful campsite in a forest of ferns.

WILD OAK

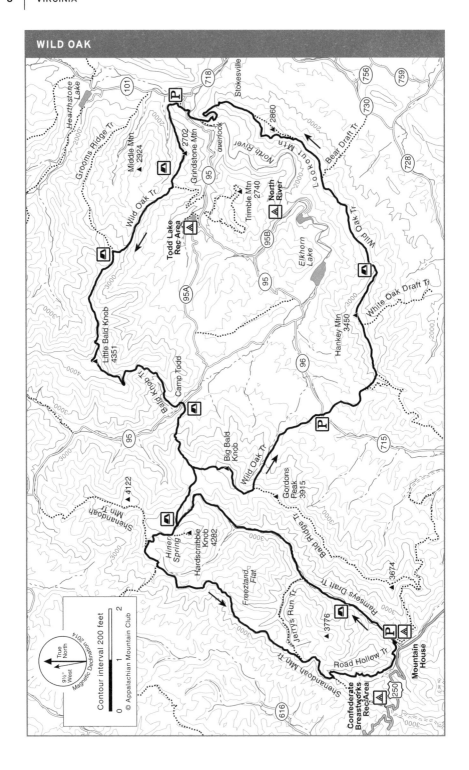

Lookout Mountain (15.3/3,061/38° 18.763' N, 79° 13.735' W). Several wildlife clearings along the broad back of this mountain offer good opportunities for camping. These sites are dry, so you'll have to carry in plenty of water.

Grindstone Mountain (24.6/2,434/38° 22.137' N, 79° 11.412' W). There are a couple of narrow sites along Grindstone Mountain's ridgeline, and there's enough (almost) flat ground where the trail from Grooms Ridge joins so that you can camp there (26.7/3,326). There is also space atop Little Bald Knob (29.3/4,351). This entire 10-mile stretch of trail, from North River to Camp Todd, is dry, so plan accordingly.

Camp Todd (32.3/2,350/38° 22.151' N, 79° 16.412' W). After crossing the North River in Horse Trough Hollow, there are a number of unofficial campsites surrounding the intersection of Wild Oak Trail and Forest Road 95. This is Camp Todd. The campsites are big and broad, and the proximity to North River is tempting, but these sites are close to the road and are sometimes used for weekend parties.

HIKE DESCRIPTION

From the parking lot, begin walking north on Ramseys Draft Trail. Over the next 6.2 miles (about 1,600 feet of gain), you'll pass through a Wilderness renowned for its ruggedness and for the remnants of old-growth forests that still stand in the draft's higher reaches.

The trail flirts on and off with the ancient remnant of a forest road, as you cross and recross the stream. Past the intersection with Jerrys Run (2.3/2,552), the gully narrows and closes in on the trail. Soon, the trail steepens and climbs for Hiner Spring (6.2/3,986), a broad area with several fine camping sites.

For the next mile and a half, you'll be using the Hiner Spring Trail to link up with the Wild Oak Trail. Just as you enter Hiner Spring, bear sharply to the right and cross the creek (one last time!). Walk gently downhill through a rhodendron thicket before reaching white-blazed Wild Oak Trail (7.7/3,745), which cuts a 26.2-mile circuit around the valley of the North River.

Initially, Wild Oak Trail climbs along the crest of Bald Ridge to the summit of Big Bald Knob (4,120 feet). The trail veers to the left at a rather murky pond (9.3/3,753). Do not proceed straight, as that trail continues southeasterly toward US 250 and the base of Ramseys Draft. From the pond, your route descends sharply, then more gently toward Forest Road 95, where there is a parking bay (11.4/2,325).

Here you'll begin a formidable ascent of about 1,200 feet up the flanks of Hankey Mountain (14.3/3,450/38° 19.0224' N, 79° 14.7198' W). One of three tough climbs on the trail, this bit of walking is made all the tougher by the several false summits along the way. Take your time, and you'll be rewarded by about 6 miles of gently descending terrain as Wild Oak Trail follows the broad back of Lookout Mountain. Pass a vehicle gate, a few turnoffs for access trails in the valley, and clearings where you have views of Elkhorn Lake far below.

As you approach the gorge of the North River, the trail plunges from the back of Lookout Mountain, veering left on a stretch of newly constructed trail. The footpath is rocky, so take care as you begin this descent. Use the marked overlook just before the lake (21.5/1,730) to peer down at the river. A few minutes farther on, a suspension bridge crosses North River (21.9/1,587). Fill your bottles here, as the next 10 miles of Wild Oak Trail are dry until you again reach the North River at Camp Todd.

Once you have the water you need, cross the bridge and climb a few switchbacks to reach Forest Road 101 (22.6/1,673). (Look to the right as you climb to catch a glimpse of a beautiful emerald swimming hole at the base of a large boulder in the river.) Beyond the road, you'll pass a spur trail on the right to the parking lot and the official start of Wild Oak Trail; the trail winds through a wooded area of oak and hickory. It very quickly gets serious about the 7-mile climb ahead, which leads over 2,702-foot Grindstone Mountain and then later the 4,351-foot Little Bald Knob.

As you climb, views of the Blue Ridge and valley start to open out. Wild Oak Trail intersects with Little Skidmore Trail (24.7/2,425). Turn hard right and look for the blazes. Over the next 2 miles, the trail climbs steadily to the intersection with Grooms Ridge Trail from the right (26.7/3,326). After that point, the trail widens and becomes easier walking for about a mile. The trail starts to climb again in good earnest just before the summit of Little Bald Knob—the highest point on the trail (29.3/4,351/38° 23.6339' N, 79° 15.4736' W).

As you reach the summit, Wild Oak Trail makes an easy-to-miss hairpin turn to the left. The summit itself is unremarkable (there is a viewpoint down the road), but you'll spot excellent overlooks as you begin the descent. This path winds its way through folds in the mountain and is, at times, moderately steep and rocky. Keep your eye out for the strange, large, red mushrooms that border the trail. Also, do be alert: copperheads, rattlesnakes, and black snakes sun themselves along trails in the area, especially in summer.

The descent nears its end when the sounds of the North River—and perhaps the sounds of the occasional vehicle passing—can be heard. Eventually, the trail splits, one branch (signed) continuing straight and the other bending sharply via a switchback to the right. Both are blazed white, no doubt confusing a hiker or two, but the signed path to Camp Todd is clear. Continue straight and very quickly come upon the North River (32.3/2,356). On the far side of the river,

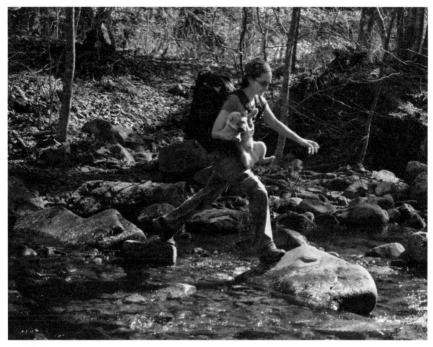

In cool weather, you will enjoy easy walking along the wide, flat trails of the Pine Barrens. A hiker—with her furry friend—looks for dry footing at one of the many crossings of Ramseys Draft.

Camp Todd, really just a few bare patches where you might pitch tents, sits astride Forest Road 95.

In the event that the North River is so swollen that crossing it might be dangerous, reascend to the intersection and take the other path with the switchback (now on your left). It will take you to Forest Road 95. Turn left, cross the river via a bridge, and hike along the road to the right bank of Camp Todd, rejoining Wild Oak Trail.

Leave Camp Todd, cross the road, and begin the sharp 1.7-mile ascent up Springhouse Ridge Trail. The trail climbs about 1,250 feet through this forest of maple, oak, hickory, and dogwood. When you reach an intersection marked by a dilapidated sign stating that the land behind it is Wilderness (33.9/3,731), you should congratulate yourself. You've completed Wild Oak Trail. Take a right, and continue about 1.5 miles back to Hiner Spring.

Backpackers often arrive at Hiner Spring, for understandable reasons, rather fatigued and unwilling to do much walking; however, the 500-foot climb to Hardscrabble Knob (about 1.2 miles roundtrip to an elevation of 4,282 feet) justifies waking up a little earlier in the morning or staying out past sunset for this out-and-back trip. Walk uphill through the Hiner Spring meadow, and turn left at the first intersection. Continue about 0.5 mile, walking through a lovely, open, fern-filled forest. When you reach the toppled remains of an old steel lookout tower, scramble up the rocks to the right of the tower to reach the summit, passing a USGS marker. The surrounding views of Elliott Knob and Bald Ridge merit a few moments of contemplation, and on a clear night, this is a wonderful spot for stargazing.

When you're ready to put Hiner Spring in the rearview mirror, you have a few choices. You could simply redescend the draft, but you probably just got your socks dry from climbing it. If you'd like to see a different side of the mountain, leave the spring by climbing over the back of the bowl. Bypass the spur trail to Hardscrabble Knob on your left, and head right along a gently descending grade. In a saddle, Tear Jacket Trail heads north and Shenandoah Mountain Trail heads south (36.2/3,754). Your path takes you southward on this exceptionally gentle and well-graded trail. Easy miles follow, with views of the Alleghenies to the right and glimpses of the valley of Ramseys Draft to your left.

You'll pass by the top of Jerrys Run (40.7/3,187), then take a left onto Road Hollow Trail (41.7/3,014), which zigs and zags its way through a number of hollows as it takes you down, almost directly, to the draft. Take a right once you reach the creek and you'll be back to your vehicle (44/2,265).

OTHER OPTIONS

With Wild Oak Trail and the various trails in the Ramseys Draft Wilderness, there are many backpacking routes that might be put together. A classic and very rewarding 16-to-18-mile loop might be hiked by simply walking a circuit around Ramseys Draft. After parking at the trailhead on US 250, climb either Bald Ridge Trail to the east of the draft or Shenandoah Mountain Trail to the west. Both will lead you to the campsite at Hiner Spring and set you up for the descent of the draft in the morning. Note that finding the trail along Bald Ridge can be an issue, but as long as you stay on the ridge, you are bound to pick it up again.

If Wild Oak Trail beckons, take advantage of the trail's several road cross-ings to set up vehicle shuttles to section-hike the trail. By leaving a vehicle at the trailhead at the North River and another at Camp Todd, you could section-hike the north or south halves of the trail, and there's also the lot just west of Hankey Mountain for a third option.

NEARBY

You'll pass through the little town of Churchville, Virginia, on your way out on US 250, and there are a few independent restaurants in town that welcome hungry hikers. If you can't find what you're looking for in Churchville, Harrisonburg on I-81 is the nearest larger town.

ADDITIONAL INFORMATION

You will find the George Washington and Jefferson National Forests' website at fs.usda.gov/gwj, and the North River Ranger District can be reached at 540-432-0187.

TRIP 3
PICTURE POSTCARD PERFECT

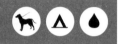

Location: George Washington and Jefferson National Forests, Virginia
Highlights: A triple crown of iconic Appalachian Trail viewpoints—
McAfee Knob, Tinker Cliffs, and Dragon's Tooth—as well as the
wilderness of the less often visited North Mountain Trail
Distance: 34.2 miles round-trip
Total Elevation Gain/Loss: 9,168 feet gain/9,168 feet loss
Trip Length: 3–4 days
Difficulty: Challenging
Recommended Maps and Other Resources:

- *Appalachian Trail Guide to Central Virginia.* Harpers Ferry, WV:
  Appalachian Trail Conservancy, 2010.
- USGS Quads: Salem, Daleville, Catawba, and Glenvar.

**Connect the dots between some of the most popular vistas of
the Appalachian Trail (AT) in southern Virginia in an ambitious
circumnavigation of Catawba River Valley near Roanoke. Few
thrills match a scramble to the top of Dragon's Tooth, with its
eagle's nest view of the surrounding mountains, but the vistas from
McAfee Knob and Tinker Cliffs come close.**

HIKE OVERVIEW

Truly a tale of two trails, this trip weaves together one of the most traveled
stretches of the AT in Virginia with the comparatively wild and seldom walked
North Mountain Trail.

Beginning where the AT crosses VA 311 just west of Roanoke and taking
you about 10 miles northbound, this section allows you to take in two of the
best viewpoints along the AT in the state—McAfee Knob and Tinker Cliffs.
Then, as the AT turns east toward I-81, head west, crossing Catawba Creek
Valley and beginning a long southbound circuit of the valley. Camp where you
can enjoy simultaneous views of the Blue Ridge to the east and Alleghenies
to the west. The southern portion of the trail brings you to Dragon's Tooth, a
third iconic view of the AT. Finally, amble through rural countryside before
following a final ridge back to the cars.

Together these two trails escort you through a wide variety of landscapes,
including the wilds of North Mountain, some of the most photographed sights

of the AT, lovely pastoral scenes in the valley, and isolated stretches of trail that are usually only enjoyed by thru-hikers. This trip is well suited to the advanced or intermediate backpacker looking to savor a weekend's taste of what the AT has to offer. It can be done in two nights, or it can easily be extended to three or four nights of backpacking.

One interesting note: the miles from Andy Lane Trail to North Mountain Trail served as part of the AT in the 1970s. While it is perhaps true that the current path of the AT in this area is more scenic, the older route has a wild and secluded feel that the well-traveled modern path lacks.

OVERNIGHT OPTIONS

Whether you do this hike as a two- or three-night trip, sequencing your campsites will require some forethought. Parts of the AT in this section have a high concentration of shelters and campsites, while other stretches of trail have comparatively few good campsites. In some other areas (Tinker Cliffs and McAfee Knob), camping is prohibited. The campsites that are available do reward the effort of reaching them, however. Do exercise good food discipline at camp, especially when you're on North Mountain Trail; this ridge is considerably wilder and more isolated than the one on which the AT runs, and wildlife encounters are that much more likely.

Catawba Mountain Shelter (2.2/2,165/37° 23.291' N, 80° 3.428' W). A rather dense concentration of AT shelter and campsite clusters within just a few miles north of the trailhead parking lot on VA 311; these include the John Springs Shelter (0.94/1,966), the Catawba Mountain Shelter (and its associated campsite), and the Campbell Shelter (and its Pig Farm Campsite; 4.7/2,625). Catawba Mountain Shelter's spring was little more than a trickle when I passed. If you have a large group, the Pig Farm Campsite may be your best bet. If you spend the night at Catawaba Mountain Shelter, consider trying to catch the sunrise at McAfee Knob, just 1.5 miles and 1,032 feet of elevation farther along the route.

Lamberts Meadow Shelter (10.6/2,108/37° 26.077' N, 79° 59.252' W). If the sun is dropping low in the western sky as you reach Scorched Earth Gap, turn right and follow the AT about 0.6 mile beyond the gap, where a shelter and its campsite await (turn off route at 10/2,562). A stream is nearby. Though Tinker Cliffs is tempting, camping is not permitted in this high-use area.

"Singed Socks" Campsite (20.6/2,898/37° 24.158' N, 80° 6.636' W). The must-have campsite for this trip. The ridgeline along North Mountain Trail may be dry, narrow, and rarely flat, but be patient. Just a few yards past the intersection with Grouse Trail, a built-up fire ring and flat spots for two or three

tents are on the left. From this site, you can see views of the ridges to your east (McAfee Knob) and west while sitting comfortably at the fire ring. Sunsets here can be spectacular in the right conditions. Exercise particularly good food discipline here—this ridge is considerably wilder and more isolated than its neighbors. The name "Singed Socks" derives from an unfortunate failed effort to dry a pair of damp socks.

Lost Spectacles Gap (25.7/2,508/37° 21.950' N, 80° 9.993' W). This may be the best camping location in the southern section of the trip. Dragon's Tooth Trail and the AT intersect in a broad saddle just north of Dragon's Tooth. This saddle is named Lost Spectacles Gap for a local trail maintainer and scout who lost his eyewear there. It is dry, so plan to carry water up from McAfee Run.

If you're doing this trip in two nights, camp at Catawba Mountain Shelter and then Singed Socks campsite—really, the most beautiful campsite on the trail. Your splits would be approximately 2.1–18.3–13.6. If you're walking it with three campsites, consider visiting McAfee Knob and Tinker Cliffs and spending the night at the Lambert Meadows Shelter, then at Singed Socks, and then passing the final night at Lost Spectacles Gap. Your splits might be closer to 10–11–6.9–6.9.

HOW TO REACH THE TRAILHEAD

From I-81 southbound, take Exit 141 for VA 419 toward VA 311 North/Salem/ New Castle. Turn left on VA 419, and then soon thereafter, turn right on VA 311. About 5.6 miles later, you'll reach the top of the pass and see a parking lot on the left (37° 22.8017' N, 80° 5.3713' W). If you start to descend into Catawba, Virginia, you've gone too far.

HIKE DESCRIPTION

From the parking lot on VA 311, locate the white-blazed AT, which enters the lot from the south, crosses the road, and begins a traverse with a few gentle uphill sections along the southern slopes of McAfee Knob. For the first few miles of the trail, the path is big, broad, and sandy, and is obviously well used by day-hikers and weekend campers. Though the trail climbs gently from the parking lot, you'll soon be walking on mostly level ground, crossing occasional numbered bridges where the side-hilling path become a bit eroded.

After about 1 mile, the AT dips down, swings left, and you'll see the Johns Spring Shelter on the right. Another mile of easy walking takes you to the spring for the Catawba Mountain Shelter, which precedes the shelter itself and its campsite (2.2/2,165). As you approach the shelter, the trail splits, with signs pointing left to the campsite and right to the shelter.

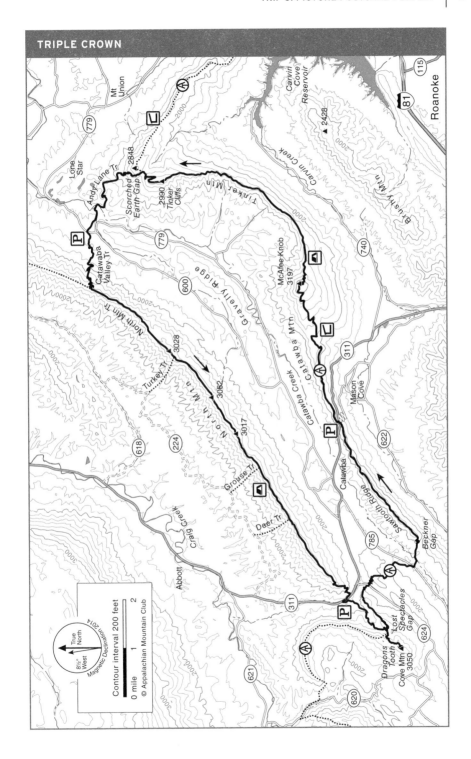

From the campsite, the AT begins a sustained, if not especially steep, 1.5-mile ascent to McAfee Knob (3.7/3,197). If you're planning on arriving at the knob's summit before daybreak, be especially conscious of the blazes as you cross a forest road near the beginning of the climb. The trail dodges sharply left, and then switchbacks right. You'll know you've almost reached the summit of McAfee when the trail becomes slabby. Do be careful if those slabs are wet, as they can be slick.

McAfee Knob is a broad summit with a number of overhanging slabs, almost as if it were designed for taking photos of intrepid hikers staring out over the ridges of Appalachia. Now is a good time to take advantage of the panorama and survey the rest of your route. On your right are Tinker Cliffs and, behind them, Scorched Earth Gap, where you'll leave the AT and descend to the valley. Directly across from you is the long ridge of North Mountain. You'll soon be walking south along the spine of this ridge and looking back at McAfee Knob. Away to the south is Dragon's Tooth.

The trail leaves McAfee Knob and descends through an area of gigantic boulders known as the Devil's Kitchen. While the devil can cook here, you can't—this attractive area along with the knob itself is off-limits for camping and campfires. After about 1 mile and about 700 feet of descent, the AT reaches the Pig Farm Campsite and Campbell Shelter where there are legal campsites aplenty (4.7/2,625). There is also a nearby spring found by following a trail to the side of the shelter, crossing a power cut, and walking down an old road. The spring may be more reliable in some seasons; when I visited, however, it was little more than a steady drip.

Heading north along the AT, the trail follows the broad back of the ridgeline over some of the easiest miles of the trip. From time to time, the path leads you over some interesting rock formations or tantalizes you with partial views, including an impressive view of Carvin Cove Reservoir. The easy walking soon comes to an end, however, as you make the 700-foot climb to Tinker Cliffs (9.1/2,919). The views will more than amply merit the energy necessary to crest this promontory, however. The trail clambers along these beautiful sandstone cliffs for about 0.5 mile, with expansive views of the Catawba Valley and North Mountain.

Once you're done taking in the views, continue north along the AT, which parallels the rocks and descends sharply along switchbacks that dart around the base of the cliffs. When you've reached Scorched Earth Gap (10/2,562), you have a decision to make. If it's late afternoon or early evening, take the right turn to continue eastward on the AT and make camp near Lambert's Meadow Shelter. If it's earlier in the day, go ahead and start the descent on yellow-blazed

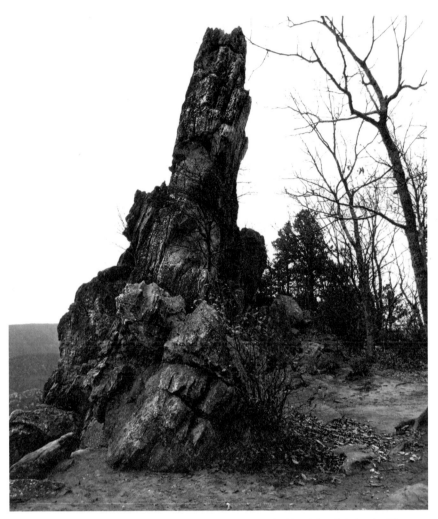

By climbing Dragon's Tooth, hikers can obtain a remarkable vista of Catawba River Valley and the Blue Ridge.

Andy Lane Trail into the Catawba Valley. Keep in mind, though, that if you decide not to stay at Lambert's Meadow, you will have to reach Catawba Creek, VA 779, and complete the climb up Catawba Valley Trail before backcountry camping will again be practical. Singed Socks is still about 10.5 miles away.

Descending Andy Lane Trail—however tough a climb it may be from the opposite direction—can be a pleasant experience in good conditions. The trail's initial descent is gradual, with switchbacks winding between the hollows. At a few points, though, the trail gives up on the switchbacks and descends straight and steep. The trail crosses an old roadbed (11.5/1,654) and bends sharply to the left. Continue the descent and soon you'll arrive at several fence crossings and the first bridge over Catawba Creek (12.2/1,334).

Here, take careful stock of your remaining water and refill your bottles as necessary. North Mountain Trail is dry, and you cannot rely on finding water again until you reach the Dragon's Tooth parking lot on VA 311, about 12 miles away. Once you've got the water you need, proceed along the trail, crossing fields, climbing stairs over fences, and clambering over another bridge. Soon you'll reach VA 785 and the parking lot there (12.9/1,476). Cross the road and keep an eye out for the informative trail sign, a little to the left. You're looking for Catawba Valley Trail, which is blazed blue. This trail climbs steadily for about 2 miles or so (the sign says 2.5 miles) from the valley to the North Mountain ridgeline, about 1,200 feet above. The trail is never especially steep and is well graded and switchedbacked in its upper reaches, but it doesn't let up on you until you reach the top. Lower down, the path follows and crosses a few streambeds before starting to climb and switchback on the face of the mountain. While the trail is blazed with bright blue plastic markers, they are few and far between. You'll need to pause from time to time to spot the next one some distance ahead in the forest.

At the top of the ridgeline, turn south off blue-blazed Catawba Valley Trail and onto yellow-blazed North Mountain Trail (14.9/2,675), which runs to VA 311 and the parking lot for Dragon's Tooth. This trail is also blazed infrequently, but the yellow blazes are always just a few steps away. It will help if you remember that the trail sticks religiously to the upper crest of the summit—it virtually never cuts around a knob or misses an opportunity for an up or a down. Just stay on the ridge, keep heading south, and pick out the occasional yellow blaze. At times, you'll have to detour around significant blowdowns, but the path is not difficult to locate on the other side.

You'll be walking southward along North Mountain Trail for about 9.5 miles. On the way, you'll pass three side trails to the right: Turkey Trail, Grouse Trail, and Deer Trail. As you work your way south, you'll have time to gaze at Tinker Cliffs and McAfee Knob, which dominate the other side of the valley, and contemplate the comparative seclusion of this trail compared to the much more popular AT. The views along this trail may not surpass those of North Mountain's more famous neighbors, but from here the ridges look apparently endless as they stretch from east to west.

You'll find Singed Socks just past North Mountain Trail's intersection with Grouse Trail (20.6/2,898). Beyond the intersection with Deer Trail, the trail follows a rockier and more knife-edged crest for a few hundred yards, then starts a sidehill descent to the left. Just when you start hearing the occasional passing vehicle far below you on VA 311, the path begins to switchback vigorously down to the road. At VA 311, turn right. You'll see a sign for the Dragon's Tooth parking lot a few hundred feet west, where there are a toilet, trash cans, and a stream from which you can treat water (24.0/1,753).

From the parking lot, the broad and well-graded, blue-blazed Dragon's Tooth Trail climbs up to where the AT passes through Lost Spectacles Gap (25.7/2,508). From here, proceed south (right) along the AT, out and back to Dragon's Tooth. It's about 0.8 mile of rocky scrambling each way; there are a few Class 3 moves for which your poles will be impediments, but as a whole the scramble is not especially difficult.

After the long leftward traverse with obstacles to climb, the trail turns rightward and climbs more steeply, with metal rungs set in the stone at two points; this last 0.3 mile to Dragon's Tooth is tough terrain for the AT. Keep your eyes out for the blazes, as they will guide you on the climb. Eventually, the trail tops out at a northerly view of the Catawba Valley. A short blue-blazed trail leads south to the rock pinnacle of the aptly named tooth.

When you reach Dragon's Tooth (26.5/3,050), you're going to want to climb it, and you should: it's a striking formation and the views from the top are well worth the effort. The climb is not especially hard, consisting really of just a single Class 3 move. If the rock is at all wet, however, stay away from this climb. The rock in this area is not at all grippy and rather frighteningly slick when wet; be cautious. If conditions are correct, walk to the front of the rock prow and turn back to its nose. You'll see a crack heading up the prow, blocked by a single boulder. It's possible to stem your way over this boulder, but the easier move involves climbing up beneath it. Once you're over this move, the big views open out. Take time to enjoy them, and get some good pictures. This is one of the best places along the AT in Virginia.

Before you leave, study the remainder of your route. From the tooth, you can easily see McAfee Knob at about 15 or 20 degrees. From its knees, you'll see a low ridge running south—Sawtooth Ridge. For the last 4 miles of this trip, you'll be walking along this ridgeline to approach the cars. If you can spot a power cut at about 50 degrees, make note: you'll soon be climbing it to reach the ridge. In total, you have about 8.0 miles remaining.

Retrace your steps to Lost Spectacles Gap (27.3/2,508), follow the AT as it climbs briefly out of the gap, and begin a long descent of about 700 feet to VA 624. If you thought you'd left the rocks behind you, think again—the path occasionally requires some scrambling and passes a few more rock structures like the tooth. One formation named Rawies Rest offers views of the Catawba

Valley to the north and east. (I had a stray thought that it should be named Dragon's Wisdom Tooth!)

Eventually, though, the AT becomes much more docile. It reaches VA 624 (28.7/1,810), climbs over another hill, crosses a creek (on a bridge), and then takes you through an area of farmlands, including a number of fence crossings. This section of trail offers a new sort of picturesque quality—it's a stretch of the AT that day-hikers rarely see. It soon crosses VA 785 (30.4/1,790) and another branch of Catawba Creek, and then climbs steeply and straight up a power cut before regaining the forests and switchbacks leading to the last ridgeline (31.3/2,329). Sawtooth Ridge provides pretty views of the surrounding ridges, but it won't let you reach the cars easily—the trail dives up and down every rocky knoll along its length, giving you a taste of what an AT thru-hiker would call "pointless ups and downs," or PUDS. The trail does become easier as you near the cars, but keep your eye out for a sharp bend that takes you down a switchback to the left, and then along some steep cliff faces. It's fairly easy to proceed straight and miss the trail.

With some perseverance, you'll soon reach the lot on VA 311 from which you began your Catawba odyssey (34.2/1,957).

OTHER OPTIONS

There are no obvious options for extending this hike, though of course you can always add extra miles along the AT, perhaps by parking a vehicle at VA 779, walking the loop as described, and then adding the section to VA 220, with a second vehicle parked near Exit 44 off I-81.

Shortening this hike is also fairly challenging. You could cut off a few miles by not visiting Dragon's Tooth and taking Boy Scout Trail to the AT from Lost Spectacles Gap, though that's not especially satisfying, given Dragon's Tooth's magnificence. It may be preferable to section-hike the trip by parking one vehicle at the McAfee Knob lot on VA 311 and another at VA 779 where it intersects Andy Lane Trail. If you're looking for a much shorter trip in this area, backpack in to the Campbell Shelter and day hike to Tinker Cliffs.

NEARBY

The culinary delights of Roanoke, Virginia, are not to be denied, especially to hungry backpackers returning, footsore and weary, from the trail. Two words: fried chicken.

ADDITIONAL INFORMATION

For additional information on the trails in this section, please contact the Glenwood-New Castle District Ranger at 540-864-5195 and the Glenwood-Pedlar District Ranger at 540-291-2188. In case of emergency, contact the Roanoke County Police and Rescue at 540-561-8036. The Roanoke Appalachian Trail Club maintains this section of the trail—see its website at ratc.org.

TRIP 4
HIGH ABOVE THE HIGHLANDS

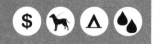

Location: Mount Rogers National Recreation Area, George Washington and Jefferson National Forests, Virginia
Highlights: Highest point in Virginia, sweeping views from the Grayson Highlands, wild ponies, and blooming rhododendron
Distance: 26.3 miles round-trip
Total Elevation Gain/Loss: 4,860 feet gain/4,860 feet loss
Trip Length: 2–3 days
Difficulty: Moderate
Recommended Maps and Other Resources:
- *Mount Rogers National Recreation Area*. National Geographic: Trails Illustrated Map, #786, 2003.
- *Appalachian Trail Guide to Southwest Virginia*, 4th ed. Ed. Thomas Vaughn. Harpers Ferry, WV: Appalachian Trail Conservancy, 2007.
- USGS Quads: Whitetop Mountain and Trout Dale.

Hiking along the balds of the Grayson Highlands, you'll find yourself surrounded by sweeping semi-alpine views of the mountains of Tennessee, North Carolina, and Virginia. Herds of wild ponies graze in the meadows. At every turn, a rocky ridge offers you the opportunity to scramble for memorably framed photographs. In season, blooming wildflowers are strewn along your path. You may be forgiven for thinking that you've died and gone to backpacker heaven. Visiting these magnificent Appalachian highlands should be high on the list of every backpacker in the region—and in the country.

HIKE OVERVIEW

Beginning at Grindstone Campground, you'll climb to reach the Grayson Highlands and Mount Rogers, and then enjoy a circuit around the area's highlights. You'll walk north on the Appalachian Trail (AT) to visit Rhododendron Gap and Wilburn Ridge, and then visit the comparatively isolated Little Wilson Creek Wilderness before returning to the AT at Scales—a place where ranchers used to gather to weigh their cattle. From this landmark, enjoy more boundless mountain views on Crest Trail before descending on Cliffside and Lewis Fork trails to your vehicle. Overall, with its moderate walking and ex-

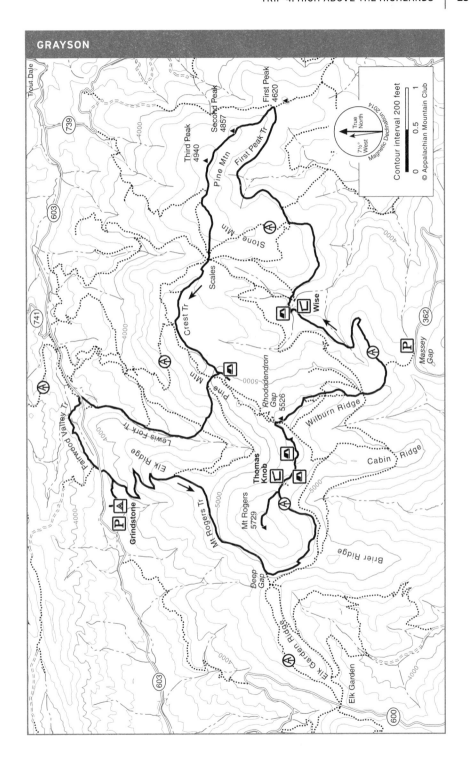

GRAYSON

ceptionally high rewards, this beautiful circuit will please both new backpackers and the most demanding, grizzled veterans.

HOW TO REACH THE TRAILHEAD

To visit the Grayson Highlands from most points in the Mid-Atlantic, you'll be spending quite a lot of time driving south on I-81. After you pass Marion, Virginia, take Exit 35 and head south on VA 107/Whitetop Road. Over the next 10 miles, this road bears several names, including CR 600. Continue south on it until you reach CR 603/Laurel Valley Road. Take a left and drive about 4.4 miles. You'll see the sign for the Grindstone Campground on your right (36° 41.2142' N, 81° 32.5631' W). Pull in and speak with the staff to make arrangements for parking your car, for a small fee.

OVERNIGHT OPTIONS

With few exceptions (such as the spur trail to the summit of Mount Rogers and the immediate vicinity of Wise Shelter), backcountry camping is allowed throughout the area without a permit. You won't hurt for wonderful campsites, but some of them can be quite popular, especially in high season. Do remember that the shelters are, first and foremost, for the use of AT thru-hikers.

Thomas Knob Shelter (7.2/5,413/36° 39.395' N, 81° 32.114' W). Located near the spur trail to Mount Rogers, this shelter is exceptionally popular and often crowded. Grab water from the spring behind the shelter, but then walk on to some of the amazing campsites a little farther north on the AT. There are quite a few, and they are big, broad, and frequented by wild ponies. One of the last ones (7.87/5,430/36° 39.1798' N, 81° 31.3238' W) also has easy access to Rhododendron Rocks, from which you can enjoy a magnificent sunset.

Wise Shelter (12.5/4,410/36° 39.24' N, 81° 29.902' W). Less popular than Thomas Knob, this typical three-sided AT shelter is located near Wilson Creek. Tenting is not permitted in the immediate vicinity of the creek, but if you follow the AT to the far bank, you'll find some good spots (12.7/4,389).

Crest Trail (21.3/5,040/36° 40.050' N, 81° 30.693' W). There is a beautiful campsite with expansive views of the highlands where Crest Trail intersects Lewis Fork Trail. This "must-have" campsite is only slightly marred by the cow and pony paddies (a disadvantage of all these free-roaming critters). Water is available at a spring a little farther along. Follow the sign into another campsite, and then pass through it to find the trickle of water (36° 39.948' N, 81° 30.795' W). If you're walking this trip in a dry month, you might want to bring your water with you, as this source could become unreliable.

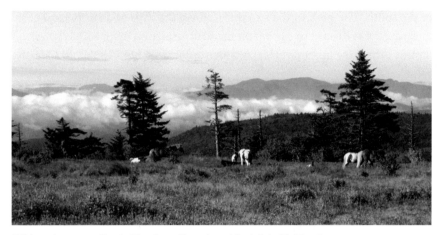

Wild ponies graze the balds of southwestern Virginia's highlands.

If you're looking for an established campsite, Grindstone Campground is an attractive destination, as are the campgrounds in Grayson State Park.

HIKE DESCRIPTION

From Grindstone Campground's overnight parking lot, begin walking back toward the campground entrance. Keep your eye out on the right for a spur trail that will take you directly to Mount Rogers Trail, just south of the trailhead. Turn (south) right when you reach the trail to begin the climb and proceed along the described route. When I visited, however, this trail was closed, so I walked out the entrance to the campground, took a right on VA 603, and walked about 0.3 mile to the trailhead on the road (0.68/3,778).

One way or another, take Mount Rogers Trail to begin your climb up to the AT. From Grindstone to the summit of Mount Rogers—the highest point in Virginia at 5,729 feet—you'll climb about 2,300 feet over about 6 miles, but you shouldn't feel daunted. Mount Rogers Trail is exceptionally well graded, with very fine footing as it switchbacks up the mountain's north face. Before long, it passes the intersection with Lewis Fork Spur Trail (2.59/4,675). The footing becomes a little rockier before the trail arrives at the intersection with the AT at Deep Gap (4.66/5,088). Be careful here as you reach the AT at the elbow of a sharp turn—the downward leading trail is headed south. You want to go north and continue uphill.

Over the next 1.35 miles, the AT traverses the southern face of Mount Rogers, gently climbing toward the open areas. Just as it reaches the spur trail leading to the mountain's summit (5.99/5,410), the balds will allow you glimpses of the mountains of North Carolina and the Smokies of Tennessee to the south. The path to the summit is about 0.5 mile and steepens slightly toward the top. Keep your eye out for the rock formation (with a USGS marker) on this otherwise unremarkable, wooded summit (6.5/5,729/36° 39.6115' N, 81° 32.68883' W).

Once you're back to the AT, continue north. The trail very quickly arrives at the Thomas Knob Shelter (7.2/5,413). Although you'll probably want to visit the spring out back, the shelter is often too crowded for comfort. Walk on for your choice of a number of very fine campsites, each with easy access to great views. Past these campsites is Rhododendron Rocks, a rocky cliff you can scramble up for views to the north (8.22/5,399). There are few finer Mid-Atlantic vistas.

Just beyond these rocks, the AT enters Rhododendron Gap, where a number of trails come together (8.76/5,471). Take careful note of this point. The AT comes in from the west and traces an inverted "C" around the highlands. Crest Trail and Pine Mountain Trail complete this circuit, making picturesque high country loops possible. As you proceed on the AT, you descend along Wilburn Ridge. At every turn, views more beautiful and more expansive than the last open out before you. Ease your way through "Fatman Squeeze" (a narrow cave), watch the wild ponies frolic in the balds, and stroll through wild gardens overlooking apparently endless mountains. Truly, this is superb walking that every backpacker in the region should know like the back of his or her hand.

When you reach the turnoff for the trailhead at Massey Gap (10.6/4,869), continue north on the AT, which will leave the balds and drop down into the drainage for the Quebec Branch of Wilson Creek. It crosses the branch on a bridge (11.7/4,660), and then descends gently along the left bank through a tunnel of rhododendron to the Wise Shelter (12.5/4,410). The trail takes a sharp left-hand turn over this burbling creek (12.7/4,641). Filling your bottles may be in order.

The AT passes a few side trails, enters the Little Wilson Creek Wilderness, and intersects with Bearpen Trail (14.2/4,641). Here, take a right on Bearpen Trail to leave the AT (and the blazes) for a quick jaunt through this less traveled part of the highlands. Bearpen Trail quickly turns into Kabel Trail. A sign warns of deep mud, but don't let that deter you. The trail runs broad and wide, follows some old road grade across the mountain, and eventually joins First Peak Trail at a little clearing near First Peak (16.3/4,526). Take a left and enjoy a few ups and downs as First Peak Trail passes over Second Peak and Third Peak. The trail then passes through a gate and into open country. The walk along the balds and into Scales (19.5/4,634), where you briefly rejoin the AT, is breathtaking and will more than make up for any mud on your shoes.

(If you don't fancy this additional loop, the walk along the AT into Scales is straightforward and also quite beautiful. You'd be cutting almost 4 miles from your route.)

As you leave Scales, climb out of the area on the unblazed Crest Trail, which first heads northwest, and then bends to the west, and finally to the southwest as it returns toward Rhododendron Gap. Broad and easy walking, Crest Trail provides views that are nearly the equal of those along Wilburn Ridge. You'll come to the intersection with Lewis Fork Trail and the campsites and nearby spring (21.3/5,040). Even if you don't spend the night, pause and explore this beautiful area.

Although you will probably regret leaving the highlands, the trip back to the car is only 5 miles. Walk northwest on Lewis Fork Trail, past the intersection with Pine Mountain Trail (22.1/4,999). Take Cliffside Trail a few yards farther along, which—true to its name—plunges off the mountain, losing altitude quickly and bringing you back to a close, but lovely, Mid-Atlantic forest. When the trail draws near to the creek, the rate of descent slows, and you'll pass through thickets of rhododendron to another intersection with ubiquitous Lewis Fork Trail (23.5/3,843). Continue straight onto this trail, which enters pastureland as it nears VA 603.

Bear right, pass through a gate, and cross the road (24.5/3,570) to gain access to Fairwood Valley Trail, which cuts through some pleasant meadows and skirts the road before delivering you to the Mount Rogers trailhead, where your trip began (25.7/3,758). Return to Grindstone Campground, walking on either he road or the spur trail, to reach your vehicle (26.3/3,707).

OTHER OPTIONS

Of course, where the AT goes, you have great opportunities for adding miles, and the Mount Rogers Recreation Area is particularly rich in side trails for you to explore. An especially fun jaunt through this area can be arranged by walking about 50 miles from the highlands into Damascus, Virginia. Not only is Damascus one of the best trail towns along the AT, but it offers a number of fun activities for the adventuresome. Consider renting a bike and cycling the Virginia Creeper Trail.

If you're looking to walk a shorter trip but still want to see plenty of the highlands, park at Massey Gap, ascend the spur trail to the AT, and then walk this loop, largely as written (skipping the additional miles in the Little Wilson Creek Wilderness by staying on the AT). Instead of descending Cliffside Trail, however, just continue on Crest Trail to Rhododendron Gap, visit Mount Rogers, and return to your car via the AT. With this route, you'll have walked a very moderate loop of about 15 miles that visits all the best scenery while avoiding the climb from Grindstone and the descent back down to VA 603.

NEARBY

In southwest Virginia, you'll be quite some distance from any large cities. Damascus is an attractive little trail town, however, and with the AT passing through, it boasts many of the services a backpacker wants. Visiting during Trail Days (May) is always fun. Marion and Abingdon, Virginia, are located along I-81 and offer the services you'd expect near the interstate.

ADDITIONAL INFORMATION

To learn more about Grayson Highlands State Park, visit its website at dcr.virginia.gov/state_parks/gra.shtml or call 276-579-7092. Additional information about the Mount Rogers National Recreation Area can be found on its website at fs.usda.gov/detail/gwj/specialplaces/?cid=stelprdb5302337, or by calling 888-265-0019. Finally, you may want to contact the Grindstone Campground (276-783-5196) to arrange for parking.

TRIP 5
I LIKE BIG RIDGES AND I CANNOT LIE

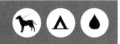

Location: George Washington and Jefferson National Forests, Virginia
Highlights: Signal Knob, Kennedy Peak, ridge walking Massanutten Mountain
Distance: 67.4 miles round-trip
Total Elevation Gain/Loss: 11,868 feet gain/11,868 feet loss
Trip Length: 3–7 days
Difficulty: Epic
Recommended Maps and Other Resources:
- Potomac Appalachian Trail Club, *Map G, Trails in the Massanutten Mountain—North Half, Signal Knob to New Market Gap, George Washington National Forest, Lee Ranger District, Virginia.*
- Potomac Appalachian Trail Club, *Guide to Massanutten Mountain Hiking Trails.* 5th ed. Vienna, VA: Potomac Appalachian Trail Club, 2008.
- USGS Quads: Toms Brook, Rileyville, Strasburg, Hamburg, and Edinburg.

Just a few miles past Shenandoah National Park and Skyline Drive—but a world apart in terms of the crowds—you'll find Massanutten Mountain, a long series of ridges running parallel to the Blue Ridge. Walking these ridges will offer you the distilled essence of the Virginia ridge ramble. Marvel at the wide open views of the North and South Forks of Shenandoah River below, the Blue Ridge to the east, the Alleghenies to the west, and—most of all—the solitude all around.

HIKE OVERVIEW

From where Massanutten Trail (MT) descends off Signal Knob and reaches VA 678 in Fort Valley, you'll walk a long, flat ellipse, hiking about 32.4 miles south to the Duncan and Strickler Knob area. Just a few miles north of US 211, you'll climb Waterfall Mountain, turn north, and return via the western ridge of Massanutten. Signal Knob—a prominence that dominates the area and was used by both sides in the Civil War—is your final highpoint and the sign that you are nearly home. While there is a fair amount of climbing and

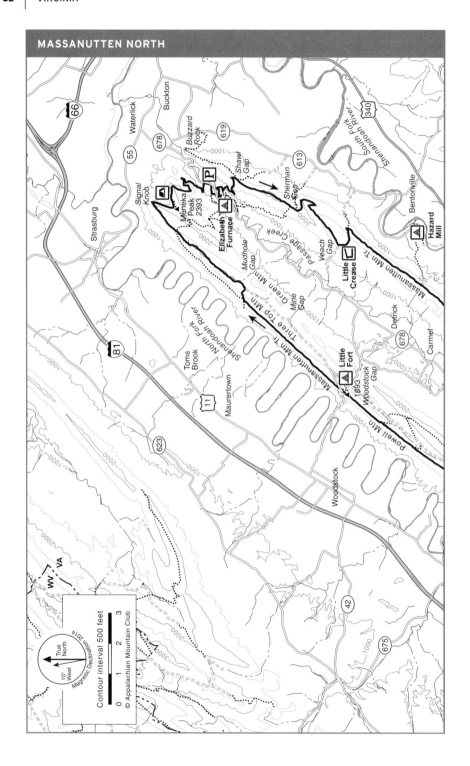

MASSANUTTEN NORTH

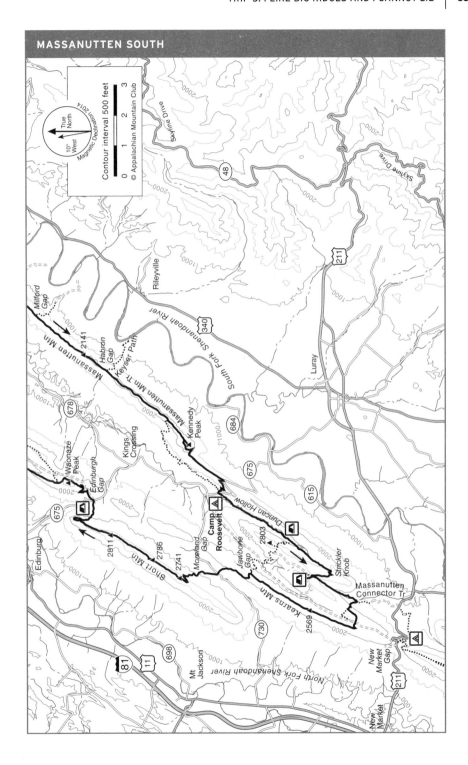

MASSANUTTEN SOUTH

descending on this trail, the long ridges mean that there is also quite a bit of flat, if sometimes rugged, walking.

Part of the appeal of walking such a big trip on Massanutten Mountain is the sense that few have preceded you. That also means, however, that the path is not always as well trod and docile as more popular trails. Even by Mid-Atlantic standards, MT is a notoriously rocky trail. Kerns Mountain, Short Mountain, Three Top Mountain, and the descent from Signal Knob will all test your ability to move over asteroid fields of jagged, uneven ground. The long north–south ridges, however, may be the purest expressions of the Virginia ridge walk and offer great rewards, with their big vistas of the Blue Ridge, the North and South Forks of the Shenandoah River, and Fort Valley itself. The ridges are narrow enough so that you'll often be enjoying views in several directions.

Besides the rough terrain, there are a few disadvantages to the trip. Water can be quite scarce for many miles, and you will be exposed to the elements, especially the sun. Plan to walk this trip in spring or fall, when the temperatures are cooler and there is water on the mountain. If you do go during a warmer season, plan your water carefully. You may very well need to cache water at key points. Always carry capacity for 4–5 liters (or more, dependent on your needs), as a dry campsite may very well be in your future.

HOW TO REACH THE TRAILHEAD

From I-66, take Exit 6 in Front Royal, Virginia, and head south on US 522 for about 1 mile. Turn right on VA 55 and drive west for about 5 miles, then turn left onto SR 678/Fort Valley Road. Enter the George Washington and Jefferson National Forests, and scope out Buzzard Rocks above you on the left. The parking lot for Signal Knob is the second lot on the right (38° 56.0388' N, 78° 19.2255' W), just as you reach the group campground.

OVERNIGHT OPTIONS

Backcountry camping is allowed through the George Washington and Jefferson National Forests. However, many of the ridgelines that characterize this route are also narrow, rocky, and quite unsuitable for camping. Almost anywhere a spot widens out, you can count on finding a small impromptu site with a fire ring, often with impressive views. Trail junctions usually have small, serviceable sites, and there are often sites near road crossings. Given the water issues that characterize this route, you'll have ample opportunities to exercise your inventiveness when it comes to planning and sequencing your campsites.

Little Crease Shelter (8.7/1,190/38° 52.175′ N, 78° 21.569′ W). This well-kept three-sided shelter in Veach Gap is located near water and features a privy, tent sites, and large fire pit. Two bunk beds in the shelter accommodate about eight backpackers.

Duncan Hollow (27.0/1,814/38° 41.576′ N, 78° 32.881′ W). By the time you cross VA 675 and reach Duncan Hollow, your bottles will likely be empty, so you'll be glad to hear water running in the hollow. There are several attractive tenting sites on the left near the intersection with blue-blazed Peach Orchard Gap Trail.

Scothorn Gap (30.0/2,460/38° 41.183′ N, 78° 34.253′ W). About 3 miles farther along MT from Duncan Hollow, you'll reach the intersection with Scothorn Gap Trail. Continue straight (west) on this yellow-blazed trail and pass a pond to see a campsite on your right. If you're worried about the pond water, descend a little along Big Run on MT and you'll have ample running water.

Edinburgh Gap (46.2/1,841/38° 47.390′ N, 78° 31.800′ W). As MT descends into Edinburgh Gap, there is a white blaze marking a tenting site. The nearby creek is seasonal, but there is a reliable piped spring about 0.5 mile east along VA 675. If you were going to cache supplies somewhere along MT, Edinburgh Gap might be the spot.

Little Fort Recreation Area (54.2/1,825/38° 52.291′ N, 78° 26.903′ W). If you reach Woodstock Gap and are in need of a place to spend the night, there is a small campsite nearby. From the pink-blazed trail that services Woodstock Tower, descend on the white-blazed trail to reach the campground, which has eleven sites open year-round (38° 52.026′ N, 78° 26.666′ W). There is no fee and no drinking water, but Peters Mill Run is nearby.

Little Passage Creek (59.3/1,240/38° 55.417′ N, 78° 22.712′ W). After you wave good-bye to Tuscarora Trail on Three Top Mountain, descend to Mudhole Gap, where campsites abound along Little Passage Creek.

Signal Knob (64.2/2,239/38° 57.148′ N, 78° 19.737′ W). As you walk eastward from Signal Knob Overlook, pass the turnoff for white-blazed Meneka Peak Trail. Beyond it, you'll soon spot a few small campsites. They're dry, but the views are remarkable.

HIKE DESCRIPTION

Locate the spur trail at the south end of the parking lot. It joins up with the orange-blazed MT, which has bypassed the lot to the west. Walk south for about 0.5 mile, skirting VA 678 on the left. The trail will intersect with blue-blazed Tuscarora Trail, which heads right to West Virginia (0.5/883). You'll turn left

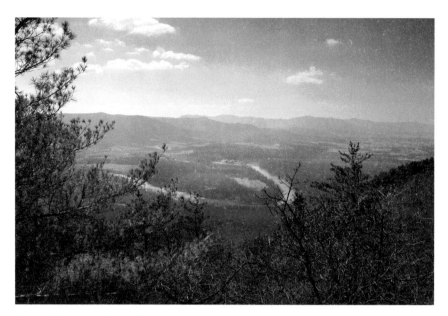

Beneath the east ridge of the Massanutten Mountains, the Shenandoah River twists its way through idyllic Virginia countryside.

onto a combined blue-and-orange-blazed trail that descends quickly, crosses VA 678, and cuts through the Elizabeth Furnace Campground (1.0/746).

For a spell, MT coincides with Pig Iron and Charcoal interpretive trails, but very soon the path steepens and begins the long and sometimes steep climb to Shawl Gap, the first of many such gaps you'll pass as you proceed south along the palisades of Massanutten Mountain (3.35/1,686). At the white-blazed trail from Buzzard Rocks that comes in on your left, turn right, following the blue-and-orange-blazed trail as it climbs an additional few hundred feet before topping out on the ridgeline. About 2 miles of ridge walking will take you to Sherman Gap (5.5/1,934), where a pink-blazed trail intersects from the right, combines for a stretch (yes, pink, orange, and blue blazes!), and then exits left. Continue south.

Climb about 300 feet past Sherman Gap, where you'll enjoy some big views of the Shenandoah. After a sharp right turn (6.7/1,783), the trail begins a steady descent into Veach Gap, with an unreliable creek on your left. Eventually, you'll hear water, and MT intersects with yellow-blazed Veach Gap Trail on the right. Continue straight, rock-hopping over Mill Run to find the Little Crease Shelter (8.7/1,190). Fill your bottles here, as this is the last reliable source of water for about 16 miles, until you reach Duncan Hollow.

When you're ready to walk on, climb about 600 feet to rejoin the ridgeline along a very old road bed. This road was constructed during the Revolutionary War, when General Washington feared that the Continental Army might be forced to retreat to Fort Valley. Once you reach the top of the ridge, the Tuscarora Trail bears east and descends the road grade, heading toward the Appalachian Trail atop the Blue Ridge (9.7/1,856).

Your route takes you south on a path that is now orange-blazed only, and you'll cover the miles swiftly as the trail makes a beeline for Kennedy Peak. Before it reaches Milford Gap, the trail splits in two, with the official blazed branch sidehilling along the eastern flank of the mountain. Big views to the east and the west ensue as you reach Milford Gap (12.8/1,756), Indian Grave Trail (14.5/1,926), Habron Gap (18.2/2,113), and Jacks Notch, each with trails leading off the ridge. Don't be distracted; Kennedy Peak looms before you. When MT bends right to go around it, instead climb the white-blazed spur trail to reach the observation tower and sweeping views of the Shenandoah river valleys (20.8/2,540/38° 44.5171' N, 78° 29.2607' W).

Once you rejoin MT, the walk down from Kennedy Peak is relaxed, coinciding with a road that is open to ATV traffic (you'll spot some passable campsites if you don't intend to reach Duncan Hollow right away). Soon the trail meets up with VA 675 at Edith Gap (23.4/1,849). To the left is an opening where hang gliders sometimes fly. Turn sharply right on the road, locate the next orange blaze, and leave the road to the right. MT descends gently through the forest, crossing a couple of power line cuts until it reaches a few outbuildings and VA 675 again (24.3/1,334). The Camp Roosevelt picnic area is just to the west along VA 675 and, in summer, you'll be able to fill your bottles there.

After you cross VA 675, you'll be in Duncan Hollow. MT soon winds its way south and eventually leads you across a very reliable creek. For the next 3 miles, MT ascends along the right side of this creek, and you'll have ample opportunity to rehydrate and fill your bottles. At the intersection with Peach Orchard Gap Trail (27.0/1,814)—if you have the time—consider leaving MT to ascend to the saddle, adding an extra 2 miles round-trip. The scramble up to the summit of Duncan Knob offers memorable views, and you can camp below the knob.

After this intersection, MT continues south, climbing more steeply and eventually switching back over the crest of Middle Mountain. (Again, if time permits, consider bushwhacking out and back to Strickler Knob, which offers views to the south; this out-and-back would add about 1.5 miles to your trip.) MT quickly drops down to Scothorn Gap and Scothorn Gap Trail (30.0/2,460), where it turns left and descends Big Run southerly. Camping is straight ahead on the Scothorn Run Trail.

The descent of Big Run is rocky and watery, as MT alternately sidehills up high above the creek and then dives down for a crossing. At the bottom, MT meets white-blazed Massanutten Connector Trail coming in from US 211 to the south (32.4/1,617). Pause to shed a few layers and make sure your bottles are topped off, and then turn right and begin the toughest ascent on the trip: the 800 feet up Waterfall Mountain. Though stout, the ascent is blissfully direct, and the trail crests the mountain along open and flat land before crossing Crisman Road (32.5/2,322).

Just past the road, MT turns north and begins traversing the long westward ridges heading back to Signal Knob. For the first 4 miles, walk along Kerns Mountain where the trail continually flirts with the ridgeline over some exceptionally broken ground. Then at the four-way intersection at Jawbone Gap (37.7/2,402), drop your pack and clamber an extra 0.1 mile up to the rocky promontory for the view. From there, the descent to Moreland Gap Road is gentle (39.2/1,907). After crossing Moreland Gap Road, the trail shadows Edinburgh Gap Road through the woods on the right, crosses it, and then climbs steeply to the crest of Short Mountain (40.9/2,747).

The next few miles are treacherous walking before the trail begins a circuitous descent into Edinburgh Gap (46.2/1,841). In the gap, turn left onto VA 374 very briefly, pass the ATV parking on the right, and cross VA 675 (46.5/1,709). On the other side of the road, begin the climb up Waonaze Peak, but before you leave this gap, consider carefully if you need to detour to the spring about 0.5 mile east on VA 675. The next reliable water on the trail is 13 miles ahead, at Little Passage Creek.

Once you summit Waonaze Peak (48.1/2,705), you'll enjoy about 6 miles of fairly flat ridge walking along Powell Mountain. This stretch is one of the most pleasant of the trip, with many views of the mountains to the west. Pass Bear Trap Trail, 7-Bar None Trail, and Lupton Trail on the right, and soon arrive at Woodstock Gap and the observation tower (54.2/1,825).

Easy miles follow Woodstock Gap as the trail continues north along the ridge of Three Top Mountain. MT passes Mine Gap Trail, intersects briefly with Tuscarora Trail (58.6/1,712), and then descends to Mudhole Gap (59.4/1,204), where it turns north for about 4 miles along a service road that parallels Little Passage Creek. The road ascends gently past an artificially constructed pond, passes yet another intersection with Tuscarora Trail, and grows steep as it climbs to the summit of Signal Knob (63.3/2106), the northernmost point on Massanutten Mountain and one of the best viewpoints in the area.

Once you've drunk your fill of this view, descend 4 miles to the end of the trip, passing Meneka Peak Trail and then overlooks of Fort Valley (65.4/1,794) and Buzzard Rocks (66.0/1,518). Unfortunately, this descent crosses a number of rock fall areas, which offer very treacherous footing. Once you have passed the Buzzard Rocks viewpoint, the trail approaches the level of the road, and eventually turns left to follow a gully. The Signal Knob parking lot is a few tenths of a mile beyond (67.4/756).

OTHER OPTIONS

You probably won't want to add miles to this epic, but if you're looking to change things up, consider starting and finishing at the Buzzard Rocks parking lot on VA 619. This would add a few miles to your route and allow you to visit the knife's edge ridge of the rocks themselves.

If you're interested in cutting this long trip down to size, section-hike the eastern and western ridges independently, parking a shuttle vehicle at US 211 and the Signal Knob parking lot. Each of these ridges can effectively be cut in half by using Milford Gap Trail on the east side or Edinburgh Gap on the west. Another option is backpacking a fine loop in the south by walking north from US 211 on white-blazed Massanutten Connector Trail and then exploring the Duncan Knob and Strickler Knob area. A number of connector trails facilitate trips in this area, and the knobs both feature great views and some rock scrambling.

NEARBY

The Signal Knob trailhead is just a few miles outside both Strasburg and Front Royal, Virginia, where there are the usual array of businesses serving travelers along the interstates and a number of independent restaurants as well. If you happen to be using the trailheads on US 211, there are several local restaurants nearby, and New Market, Virginia, is not far.

ADDITIONAL INFORMATION

For additional information, contact the Lee Ranger District of the George Washington and Jefferson National Forests at 540-984-4101. The website is fs.usda.gov/gwj.

TRIP 6
THE RAGGED EDGE

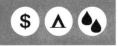

Location: Shenandoah National Park, Virginia
Highlights: Waterfalls of Cedar Run, views from the summits of
Hawksbill Mountain and Stony Man, and the classic scramble along
the ridgeline of Old Rag
Distance: 24.2 miles round-trip
Total Elevation Gain/Loss: 7,058 feet gain/7,058 feet loss
Trip Length: 2–3 days
Difficulty: Challenging
Recommended Maps and Other Resources:
- Potomac Appalachian Trail Club, *Map 10, Appalachian Trail and
  other Trails in the Shenandoah National Park, Central District.*
- Potomac Appalachian Trail Club, *Appalachian Trail Guide to
  Shenandoah National Park, With Side Trails.* 14th ed. Vienna, VA:
  Potomac Appalachian Trail Club, 2012.
- USGS Quads: Big Meadows and Old Rag.

**If you were going to do only one backpacking trip in Shenandoah
National Park, this is the one you should choose. While this 24-
mile trip is far from easy, the route visits one park highlight after
another, sometimes in such quick succession that the scenery and
the climbs may be equally likely to take your breath away. From big
views from Stony Man (4,011), Hawksbill Mountain (4,050), and
Old Rag (3,268), to the scrambling challenges of the classic Ridge
Trail, to the waterfalls of Cedar Run, and the descent through
Virginia history in Nicholson Hollow, this Blue Ridge hike has a lot
to offer an ambitious hiker.**

HIKE OVERVIEW

From the base of the park, this route takes you up Cedar Run to the park's
highest point at Hawksbill Mountain, then north along the Appalachian Trail
(AT) to Stony Man. From there you'll descend Nicholson Hollow and pitch
camp to get an early start on Old Rag. If there's any downside to the adrenaline
rush of the rocky scramble over Old Rag's ridgeline and summit, it's that the
hike is so popular. If you day hike this mountain, you're likely to find yourself
up there with a few thousand of your best friends, parking in Old Rag's muddy

cow pasture overflow lot and standing in lines a few dozen deep at some of the more challenging obstacles. It may make you want to be somewhere less crowded—like maybe Manhattan. As a backpacker, you're equipped to counter this madness by pitching your tent within 30 minutes of the Ridge Trail. With an early start from Nicholson Hollow, you can enjoy the summit while most day-hikers are just rolling into the parking lot.

HOW TO REACH THE TRAILHEAD
Heading west from Washington, D.C., on I-66, take Exit 43A and merge onto US 29 South, which will take you southeast to Warrenton. Once in Warrenton, you'll bear right onto US 211, which heads to Sperryville, Thornton Gap, and the center of the park. You'll arrive in Sperryville after about 27 miles. Turn left onto US 522 South, pass over a creek, and then turn left again in front of the restaurants in the center of town. In just under 1 mile, turn right on VA 231, which you'll follow for about 10 miles, passing the signs for Old Rag. Turn right on Etlan Road/VA 643—there is a brown sign directing you to the White Oak Canyon parking lot. After about 4 miles, turn right onto the Weakley Hollow Road and follow it for about 3 miles. Turn left into the parking lot (38° 32.2874' N, 78° 20.8731' W).

OVERNIGHT OPTIONS
There are quite a few lovely backcountry camping spots in Shenandoah National Park, but they are closely regulated by the park service. You are required to obtain a backcountry camping permit, either by mail or by visiting one the park's fee stations. The closest fee station for this trip is the one located at the Old Rag parking lot near Nethers. There are also self-registration kiosks at park entrances.

The National Park Service maintains two online videos about how to back-country camp in Shenandoah National Park (nps.gov/shen/planyourvisit/campbc.htm). Study them before you go, but here are the highlights.

- Remember that you cannot camp along the ridgeline of Old Rag or most of the summits in the park.
- No campfires are allowed in the backcountry.
- Be sure to hang a bear line or use canisters.

The name of the game for this trip is to reach Nicholson Hollow, and camp as near to the base of the hollow as you can so that you can reach the Ridge Trail as early as possible.

Rock Spring Hut (5.1/3,500/38° 33.212' N, 78° 24.498' W). If reaching Nicholson Hollow in a day seems too much, from the Salamander Trail's intersec-

CENTRAL SHENANDOAH

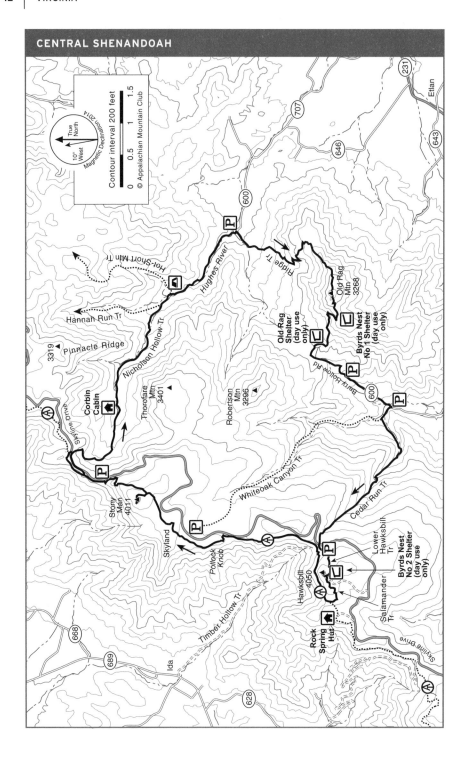

Contour interval 200 feet

© Appalachian Mountain Club

Magnetic Declination 2014

10°
West

True
North

0   0.5   1   1.5

tion with the AT (4.8/3,656), turn south and walk about 0.3 mile to this AT shelter with a spring and tent sites. Using this shelter to walk a three-day trip will enable you to hike splits of 5.1–11.5–8.2.

Corbin Cabin (13.3/2,089/38° 36.124' N, 78° 20.696' W). The Potomac Appalachian Trail Club (PATC) maintains this and a number of well-positioned cabins throughout the region. Open to the public, the Corbin Cabin is located in a particularly bucolic spot 13.3 miles from the trailhead and just about 1.6 miles along the Nicholson Hollow Trail from the AT and Skyline Drive. The cabin accommodates twelve and costs $30–45 per night; you'll need to reserve beds well ahead of time with PATC at 703-242-0315.

Intersection of Hot-Short Mountain and Nicholson Hollow Trails (15.8/1,217/38° 35.252' N, 78° 18.706' W). These are the plum campsites for those hoping to get an early start. As you're descending along Nicholson Hollow Trail with the creek on your right, you'll pass the trail marker for Hannah Run Trail (15.4/1,300) and then, shortly thereafter, the marker for the Hot-Short Mountain Trail (15.8/1,240). Immediately after you pass this sign, look to your left and you'll find a good stretch of flat ground with a number of spots for shelters. You'll have to get off the trail a bit to find them. The site's main advantage is that it is as close as you can legally camp to the beginning of Old Rag's famed Ridge Trail.

HIKE DESCRIPTION

Do not underestimate the difficulty of the ascent that begins this route, as you'll start at the base of the Shenandoah (1,160) and reach Hawksbill Mountain (at 4,050 feet, the highest point in the park) in about 4 miles. Most Shenandoah veterans would consider this climb one of the park's toughest.

As you leave the White Oak Canyon parking lot, take the blue-blazed trail. It quickly crosses a metal bridge over a creek, and then reaches a trail marker (0.3/1,153). Take the left fork for Cedar Run Trail. After a few tenths of a mile, the trail climbs quickly up to a connector trail (your last chance to end up in the wrong hollow). Stay left.

Cross the creek, and pay attention as the trail starts to climb much more aggressively. By turns, the trail will climb at a very sharp grade, riding high up the canyon walls, and then level off for a few feet as it pulls even with a swimming hole, a waterslide, or a particularly beautiful fall. Take the time to enjoy these beautiful spots, as each one is usually followed by another lung-busting, thigh-burning spurt of climbing.

Though the climb never truly relents, the toughest sections are behind you when the path crosses to the right of the creek. The uphill walking contin-

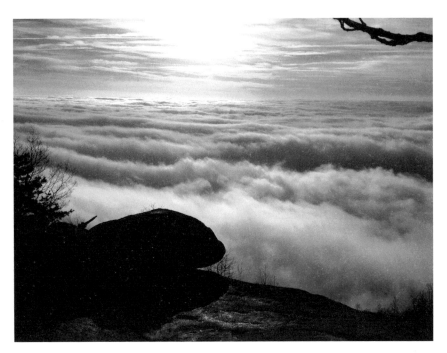

A sea of clouds washes against Old Rag's distinctively jagged ridgeline.

ues, but now through a boulder-strewn forest that opens out gradually. Stop and get water before you leave the creek bed—the ridgeline has some water sources, but it's better to be safe than sorry.

Once you reach the parking lot on Skyline Drive (3.2/3,362), you'll cross the drive, take the Lower Hawksbill Trail, and begin climbing Hawksbill Mountain. Not nearly as steep as Cedar Run Trail, this well-traveled footpath will soon bring you to the summit (4.0/4,050/38° 33.315' N, 78° 23.7092' W). The trail emerges into a clearing beside a shelter. Drink in the views of Massanutten Mountain and the Alleghenies westward, and then walk about 50 yards to the stone observation desk at the summit; this 360-degree view is one of the finest in Virginia. On a mild day, this is a wonderful spot to sun yourself on the rocks, relax, have lunch, or just enjoy the beautiful vista you've worked so hard to reach.

Hawksbill Mountain also affords you a hawk's eye view of the rest of your path through the Shenandoah. With your map in hand, let your eye follow Skyline Drive to the north where it meets Skyland; the AT follows this route closely before a brief climb to the rocky bluff of Stony Man. Beyond this mountain, the AT meets up with the Nicholson Hollow Trail, which will take you down to the east foundation of the Blue Ridge and the foot of Old

Rag. This distinctive mountain, with its ragged ridgeline, is glaring at you challengingly from the east.

To continue on, head back past the shelter to take Salamander Trail, which makes its way to the AT. Pay attention to trail markers here, as there are trails leading down to a few other parking lots for Hawksbill to the south. The blue-blazed Salamander Trail descends about 400 feet vertically down the mountain before it rejoins the white-blazed AT at a very sharp angle (4.8/3,656). Turn right to head north.

For the next mile, you'll walk on the north side of Hawksbill. Once you reach the eastern face of the mountain in Hawksbill Gap, there is a spring to the left of the AT (a trail sign marks the spot; 5.8/3,335). From the spring, the AT heads north, staying relatively flat and sticking fairly close to Skyline Drive, though it does diverge in places. Enjoy the views westward and periodically look back toward Hawksbill, which at times looms up as an impressive peak from some of the hollows. You'll pass the Crescent Rock Overlook (6.2/3,415), and the Timber Hollow Overlook (7.1/3,328), and then the trail climbs up Pollock Knob before entering Skyland—you'll know you're almost there when the AT comes up against the side of a fence.

The AT weaves its way gently through Skyland and emerges from the forest's north side to cross into the parking lot (8.9/3,695) that most day-hikers use to visit Stony Man's vista. Continue north on the combined AT–Stony Man Trail, which is blazed white and blue. In less than 1 mile, you'll reach an intersection (9.3/3,842) where the AT heads off to the right while the blue-blazed trail climbs gently about a quarter-mile to reach the summit of Stony Man (9.6/4,011/38° 35.8846' N, 78° 22.3556' W). If you time your arrival right, you can watch the sunset from here, though the view of Shenandoah is gorgeous any time of day.

With your camera doubtless full of pictures and your heart full of compassion for those who only ever see these views from their cars, continue on. From its intersection with the Stony Man Trail, the AT descends a little, eventually treating you to another fine view at Little Stony Man (10.5/3,566). Switchbacks lead down toward Skyline Drive at the Stony Man Overlook. In Hughes River Gap, you'll come upon an intersection with the blue-blazed Nicholson Hollow Trail (11.9/3,075). Turn right, cross Skyline Drive, and begin a 5.5-mile descent along the Hughes River.

Your descent on Nicholson Hollow Trail gives up most of the elevation you gained climbing out of Cedar Run (about 2,000 feet lost over 5.5 miles). With a careful eye, you can spot the remnants of old buildings along the trail, including a foundation built by Aaron Nicholson, after whom the hollow and the trail are now named. When the park was created in the 1930s, Virginia displaced 500 families from this hollow and areas like it to stitch together the protected land that comprises Shenandoah National Park today. At the time, many regarded this act as almost humanitarian intervention to bring civilization to these "hillbillies," but recent research has provided a more nuanced perspective. (For those interested in learning more of the history of Shenandoah National Park and the people who once lived here, the National Park Service has an interesting article devoted to this topic at nps.gov/shen/historyculture/displaced.htm.)

Nicholson Hollow Trail descends steeply from the AT at first—about 800 feet over the first mile—but the trail levels out. As you reach the bottom of the hollow, you'll hear the sounds of Hughes River, pass Indian Run Trail on your right, and cross the river once before reaching Corbin Cabin (13.5/2,076). After the cabin, the walking stays fairly flat and level. Cross to the left bank the river again (great care has been taken to position rocks for hopping), and pass turnoffs for the Hannah Run Trail as well as the Hot-Short Mountain Trail (16/1,222). At this intersection is a turnoff for a campsite that serves as an excellent jumping-off spot for the next morning.

At this point, you're no more than about 1.5 miles from Weakley Hollow Fire Road, and beyond it lies the classic climb of Old Rag via the Ridge Trail. Follow the Nicholson Hollow Trail as it leaves the park. Turn right onto Weakley Hollow Fire Road (17.5/934). The blue-blazed Ridge Trail is just about 0.3 mile up the road (17.8/1,072).

The journey over Old Rag divides neatly into three segments—the 1,700-foot to the ridgeline, the rocky scramble to the summit, and the descent to rejoin the Weakley Fire Road. As you leave the trailhead, the Ridge Trail climbs steadily through an open stretch of forest. Soon, it reaches the base of the ridge and switchbacks many times, more steeply. In the final few hundred feet of this ascent, the trail becomes rocky and quite steep, with slabs and steps guiding you up the mountain.

The scramble to the summit is short, rugged, and exhilarating. At times, it requires hand-over-hand climbing over its 600-foot elevation gain. Keep an eye out for the blue blazes; the route over the obstacles is not always obvious.

A few points of the scramble merit individual mention. The first challenge is a rocky slot that invites you either to crawl along a shelf to the left or climb up a split in the center (20.0/2,707). At this point, you have just less than 1 mile to the summit. Another early obstacle is a crack into which you have to lower yourself. If you sit on the edge, you can spot a few convenient footholds. Once you reach the bottom of the crack, walk along it and climb out to the left. Edge along the shelf.

The crux of the route comes after a few slabs. The trail takes a sharp right, leading you to a rock chimney that requires some climbing. Though a single hiker with a full pack can climb it alone, it's nice to be with a buddy here, as two people can overcome this section more easily.

Once you're beyond the chimney, the obstacles become easier—just a few more boulders before the sign marking the summit (20.8/3,291/38° 33.1041' N, 78° 18.8603' W).

The descent from the mountaintop is straightforward enough. A steep, switch-backed descent takes you down 436 feet to the shoulder of the mountain and Byrds Nest Shelter (21.4/2,855). A second descent switchbacks down into the hollow and eventually turns into a long, leftward traverse to the Old Rag Shelter (22.3/2,114). Only a few hundred yards of a forest road are left before Weakley Hollow Road.

Once you reach the Weakley Hollow Road (22.6/1,914), you'll take a left for a walk along a gently descending forest road. After about 1 mile, you'll leave the park at the Berry Hollow parking lot. A mile farther along, past a few houses, you'll return to the White Oak Canyon parking lot on the right (24.2/1,104).

OTHER OPTIONS

If you want to walk this trip over a three-day weekend, use the Rock Spring shelter south of Hawksbill Mountain on the AT, as noted in Overnight Options. If you're looking to extend your trip, you have quite a few options in Shenandoah National Park or along the AT. The two nearby highlights include White Oak Canyon (often hiked as a day hike with Cedar Run Trail) and Mount Robertson, which enjoys a view every bit as gorgeous as Old Rag's, but with virtually no crowds and no scrambling. Incorporating either into this trip will require some convoluted routing, but both are definitely worth the trouble. The campsite atop Mount Robertson is about as good as it gets, if you have an extra night.

NEARBY

Sperryville has a few local businesses that merit a visit (including a whisky distillery!), but if you're looking for a diner, pub, grocery store, or outdoors store, however, your best bet is Warrenton. As you drive out along US 211, keep your eyes peeled, as there are also a few wineries to visit.

ADDITIONAL INFORMATION

If an emergency occurs while you are in Shenandoah National Park, call 800-732-0911. To learn about the park, call 540-999-3500 or visit nps.gov/shen/.

TRIP 7
GO BIG (RUN) OR GO HOME

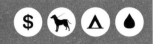

Location: Shenandoah National Park, Virginia
Highlights: The isolation of Big Run; excellent vistas from Blackrock, Brown Mountain, and Rockytop; and the waterfalls of Jones Run and Doyles River
Distance: 38.6 miles round-trip
Total Elevation Gain/Loss: 10,149 feet gain/10,149 feet loss
Trip Length: 2–5 days
Difficulty: Strenuous
Recommended Maps and Other Resources:
- Potomac Appalachian Trail Club, *Map 11, Appalachian Trail and other Trails in the Shenandoah National Park, South District.*
- Potomac Appalachian Trail Club, *Appalachian Trail Guide to Shenandoah National Park, With Side Trails.* 14th ed. Vienna, VA: Potomac Appalachian Trail Club, 2012.
- USGS Quads: Browns Cove, Crimora, Grottoes, and McGaheysville.

The southern Shenandoah may be about as close to a backpacker's paradise as you can get just two hours from the Beltway. The trails are less crowded than the northern and central districts, and limited access to Big Run's watershed means that some of the most impressive sights can best be reached by backpackers. The list of highlights is long and includes Rockytop, Big Run, Jones Run, Doyles River, Brown Mountain, and Blackrock. And, if you time your trip right, the swimming holes are superb. Walk these 38.6 miles, and you'll be eager to return to explore other trails along this circuit!

HIKE OVERVIEW

The first part of your journey will take you along Jones Run and Doyles River, with arguably the most beautiful waterfalls in Virginia. Given how renowned these easily reached trails are, you'll likely have some company until you pass the Loft Mountain Campground and begin walking north on the Appalachian Trail (AT). Once you reach Brown Mountain Trail, you'll leave the comparatively civilized terrain of Skyline Drive and dive into backcountry far from any roads, where flat land is a precious commodity. The western half of this loop is challenging terrain, with steep descents leading into one hollow after another (Big Run, Madison Run, and Paine Run), each of which is followed by a stiff climb. The last climb is also the best: it ends with the eagle's nest view from Blackrock, taking in virtually the entirety of your route and the westward stretch of the Appalachians.

HOW TO REACH THE TRAILHEAD

The Jones Run parking lot is located at Skyline Drive's mile 84, on the east side of the road (38° 13.805' N, 78° 43.572' W). To reach it, you may either enter the park southbound at Swift Run Gap, where US 33 crosses Skyline Drive, or northbound at Rockfish Gap, where I-64 crosses the Blue Ridge. Either way, you'll pay the park's entrance fee and collect a backcountry permit at these gates.

OVERNIGHT OPTIONS

There are quite a few lovely backcountry camping spots in Shenandoah National Park, but they are closely regulated by the park service. You are required to obtain a backcountry camping permit, either by mail or by visiting one the park's fee stations. There are also self-registration kiosks at some park entrances.

The National Park Service maintains two online videos that will educate you about how to backcountry camp in Shenandoah National Park (nps.gov/shen/planyourvisit/campbc.htm). Study them before you go. Remember that you cannot camp on most of the summits in the park. No campfires are allowed in the backcountry. Be sure to hang a bear line or use a canister.

Doyles River Cabin (4.0/2,539/38° 15.041' N, 78° 40.901' W). If you're interested in cabin camping one night, Potomac Appalachian Trail Club's (PATC) Doyles River Cabin is ideally positioned. As you climb Doyles River Trail, a spur leads off to the cabin to the right, about a quarter-mile before you reach the AT. You'll need to be a PATC member to enjoy this particular option, and you'll need to plan ahead—these cabins are popular.

Loft Mountain Campground (5.5/3,255/38° 14.922' N, 78° 40.240' W). The Loft Mountain Campground, Shenandoah's largest established site, is a good option for the footsore backpacker (5.5/3,255). The AT practically runs right through it, and you'll find luxuries like a camp store, showers, and laundry service. A camping spot costs $15 per night, and you would do well to reserve in advance. Open mid-May through October.

Big Run (15.8/1,260/38° 18.175' N, 78° 42.197' W). It's tough to beat the campsites you'll discover along Big Run Portal Trail. As you reach the end of

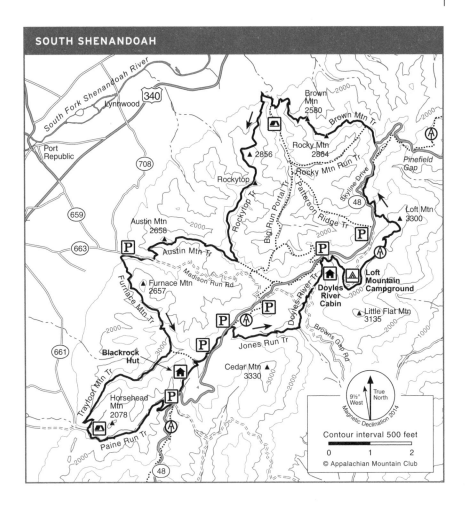

SOUTH SHENANDOAH

the descent of Brown Mountain Trail, you'll have the option of crossing Big Run via a bridge or turning left along the run. Take the left and walk along the creek. You'll soon spot smallish camping sites between the path and the water. Just before the first crossing, you'll see a number of tent sites on the left. There is more camping higher up Big Run if you're interested in exploring this lovely valley.

Paine Run (32.7/1,425/38° 11.838' N, 78° 47.271' W). Near the intersection of Paine Run Trail and Trayfoot Mountain Trail, the contour lines widen out and there are a number of pleasant camping sites with easy access to water.

Blackrock Hut (37.0/2,759/38° 12.856' N, 78° 44.576' W). This shelter is well positioned as a jumping-off point for adventures throughout the area and is quite close to the views from Blackrock itself. At 36.8 miles, take the 0.2-mile spur trail from its junction with the AT; you'll find a simple, three-sided AT shelter with a picnic table. There is a spring here, but there have been reports of it being unreliable, so carry in sufficient water.

HIKE DESCRIPTION

The parking lot and trailhead are essentially at the intersection of Jones Run Trail and the AT. Over the next 4.3 miles, you're in for quite the treat: the blue-blazed trail linking up Jones Run and Doyles River Run is arguably the best waterfall walk in Virginia. Both trails see a great deal of traffic, and though they are not precisely easy (with about 1,300 feet of descent that you then promptly regain), they are well graded and well traveled. If the weather is pleasant, expect to see plenty of other hikers.

The descent begins with a long switchback or two that then eases off and gradually descends through the more open upper reaches of the run. After about 0.5 mile, you'll cross the run. A tighter switchback brings you to the upper falls—a magnificent spot where an amphitheater of water tumbles over a rocky semicircle. The trail steepens somewhat as you continue your descent past the lower falls. You've reached the halfway point of this portion of the trail when you take a left onto Doyles River Trail (2.3/1,479).

The upper and lower falls of Doyles River are even more beautiful than those along Jones Run. When you reach the lower falls, it's definitely worth taking time to pause and get a few photos. The trail is a little steeper and rockier as it switchbacks above the waterfalls. After another 1.5 miles, pass Brown Gap Road (3.8/2,221) and continue the climb past the spur trail to Doyles River Cabin on the right (4.0/2,539). Just about 0.25 mile farther along, you'll rejoin the AT, where you'll turn north (4.3/2,626).

Initially, the AT sweeps around Big Flat Mountain and the Loft Mountain Campground (5.5/3,255); you'll see several posts pointing you to the camp-ground if you're planning to spend the night there. Pass a few rocky cliffs on the right offering views of the hollow behind you, as well as the imposing peak of Cedar Mountain (3,330), which dominates the hollow. The AT travels gently over ups and downs and intersects Frazier Discovery Trail at 7.7 miles (3,298), where there are some big westward views of Big Run's drainage.

As you walk northward, you'll leave Loft Mountain and descend about 700 feet to where the AT crosses Ivy Creek in the crook of a hollow (9.3/2,552). Fill your bottles here, as the next 6.5 miles until you reach Big Run are dry. The AT continues its gently undulating course until it reaches Ivy Creek Overlook (10.6/2,857). Pause to admire the eastward views.

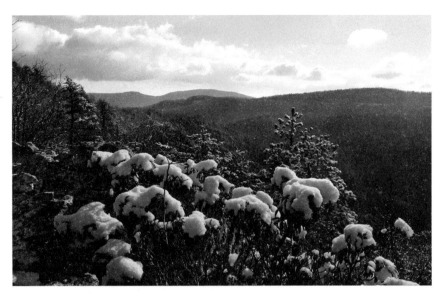

On Virginia's Blue Ridge, a spring snowfall dusts foliage along the AT.

Afterward, you'll have 0.6 mile of walking along Skyline Drive to reach the Brown Mountain Overlook and the trailhead of Brown Mountain Trail (11.2/2,854); it's curious that the two trails do not intersect.

From Brown Mountain Overlook, survey your route. You're leaving the high ridge of the AT and Skyline Drive to plunge into the hollows of the western face of the Blue Ridge. Ahead are the ridgelines of Rocky Mountain and Brown Mountain, which you'll follow west and south as they drop down into the valley of Big Run. This is the largest watershed in Shenandoah, and it dominates your left flank. Note the rocky bluffs overlooking this valley at about 10 o'clock: that is the face of Rockytop Mountain, which you'll soon be rounding for excellent views of West Virginia and the Alleghenies.

Start out on Brown Mountain Trail by descending 0.7 mile and about 500 feet down into a saddle where Rocky Mountain Run Trail intersects on the left (11.9/2,381). Head straight and regain the altitude you've lost over a couple of quick switchbacks. The trail summits Rocky Mountain (2,864/38° 17.9506' N, 78° 40.3403' W), where rock outcroppings will afford you a nice spot to take a break and admire the vistas. From here, the path begins a long and steep descent into the Big Run basin. There's no reason to rush, as you'll have many nice vistas to enjoy before you reach the intersection with Big Run and Big Run Portal Trail (15.8/1,260), where you'll probably be camping.

After an evening of exploring Big Run and perhaps, in warm weather, going for a swim in its many idyllic pools, cross the run by the bridge at the intersection with Brown Mountain Trail and walk along the south bank for about 1 mile. Soon, you'll spot the intersection with Rockytop Trail, on the left (16.9/1,338). Turn left to follow this trail.

Over the next 5.0 miles, Rockytop Trail will take you on a long but rewarding climb of the westernmost ridge boxing in the Big Run watershed. Not only does this trail offer some gorgeous views of Massanutten Mountain, the Shenandoah Valley, and the westward-stretching Alleghenies, but also the rockfalls you'll be crossing are interesting in themselves (note the long cylindrical markings in them, which are thought to be fossilized worm holes). As you start the climb, the trail switchbacks through the surrounding forest and quickly gains altitude. Soon it crosses talus slopes, which open out for the big westward views. Because this area is comparatively open for Shenandoah, bring a sun hat if you're crossing it on a warm day; the trail is also dry, so you'll want plenty of water. Swing leftward around the westward face of boulder-strewn Rockytop, drop quickly, and then pass around its southern face. From here, pass the junction with Lewis Peak Trail on the right (20/2,737), and then walk along the ridgeline, sometimes on the right and sometimes on the left, until you reach the intersection with Austin Mountain Trail (21.9/2,735). Turn right.

Walk along a fairly even ridgeline for about 2 miles before the trail plunges down about 1,300 feet to join Madison Run Fire Road (24.8/1,441). Sections of this descent are rugged, and you'll cross talus fields that will be familiar to you after Rockytop. Take a right on yellow-blazed Madison Run Trail and follow it for about 0.8 mile until you see the gate ahead and the blue-blazed Furnace Mountain Trail on your left (25.6/1,358). Cross Madison Run here, and fill your water bottles if necessary; the next water source is 7.0 miles away at Paine Run.

Over the next 3.4 miles, climb steadily about 2,000 feet to the summit of Trayfoot Mountain (3,374/38° 13.4183' N, 78° 45.0763' W). After about 1.5 miles, pass a 0.5-mile spur trail that will take you to the summit of Furnace Mountain (2,657), where there is a view. Intersect Trayfoot Mountain Trail just beneath the mountain's summit (28.7/3,177). Turning left will take you toward Blackrock and the AT; you should bear right to descend Trayfoot Mountain. You'll enjoy fine views on both sides of the upper reaches of this trail as the path follows the mountain's rather pronounced crest. Sharp turns to the left and then the right will signal that you've almost reached Paine Run, where campsites await (32.7/1,425).

Your final climb, initially along Paine Run, is perhaps not the most interesting trail in the Shenandoah, but the rewards awaiting you at Blackrock make it more than worthwhile. Take a left on Paine Run Trail and follow the yellow blazes. This trail used to be a forest road and is well graded and fairly gentle. Water and stream crossings are common at first, but as you climb the valley you'll pull away from the run. The old road will zig-zag a few times, and then intersect with Skyline Drive at Blackrock Gap (36.1/2,325). Cross the road, locate the AT, and head north.

At first, the AT sticks fairly closely to Skyline Drive, but it soon crosses the road and begins climbing steadily toward Blackrock itself. A spur trail on the right leads down about 0.25 mile to the ravine where the Blackrock Hut is located. Just a bit before the summit of Blackrock, you'll pass the beginning of Trayfoot Mountain Trail on your left. Once you reach Blackrock (37.4/3,092/38° 13.1951' N, 78° 44.4179' W), scramble to the top and enjoy one of the finest vistas in the park. Most of your route is visible beneath you: Paine Run to the southwest, Trayfoot Mountain to the west, Austin Mountain, Rockytop, and the Big Run drainage to the north. Make sure you have plenty of time to enjoy the view. You'll want to linger.

When you're ready to end your adventure, walk north along the AT. It bends around the summit and descends gradually, passing a parking lot on your left. Soon, it crosses Skyline Drive and arrives at the parking lot for Jones Run (38.6/2,765).

OTHER OPTIONS

Southern Shenandoah National Park features a wonderful network of trails, and you have multiple options for extending or shortening your trip.

If you walk south from Blackrock Gap, you'll quickly encounter Riprap Trail. Linking up this trail with Wildcat Ridge Trail will enable you to add a "lollipop" loop onto the trip as written. If you have the time, this addition is well worth it. You'll net big views from Calvary Rocks and Chimney Rock, as well as additional opportunities for backcountry camping.

Walking up Big Run Portal Trail is certainly the biggest omission from the trip, as it is one of the best trails in the Shenandoah, lined with alluring camp-sites and cooling swimming holes. If you had the time, you could easily spend an entire day (or two!) exploring this wonderful place.

For a shorter loop, close study of the map will point out a number of connector trails that could be used as cutoffs. Trayfoot Mountain Trail links up with the AT at Blackrock; Austin Mountain Trail and Patterson Ridge Trail also link up farther north. If you prefer to section-hike this trip, you could do so by using these trails to turn this trip into a two-weekend affair with north and south loops.

NEARBY

If you're returning home via I-81, downtown Harrisonburg may be your best bet for grub; Charlottesville is also nearby for those headed south and east.

ADDITIONAL INFORMATION

If an emergency occurs while you are in Shenandoah National Park, call 800-732-0911. To learn about the park, call 540-999-3500 or visit the park online at nps.gov/shen/.

2

WEST VIRGINIA

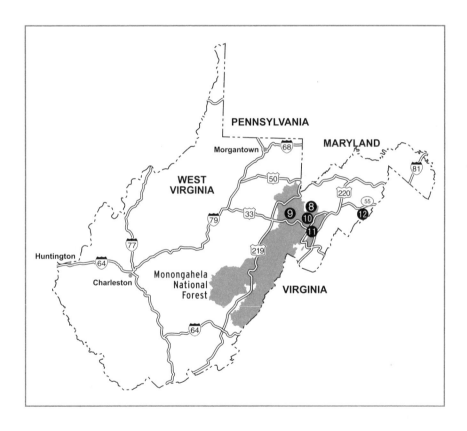

TRIP 8
HELLO, DOLLY SODS!

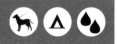

Location: Monongahela National Forest, West Virginia
Highlights: Views of the West Virginia highlands, rolling bog and heath terrain unique to the region
Distance: 24.6 miles round-trip
Total Elevation Gain/Loss: 3,793 feet gain/3,793 feet loss
Trip Length: 2–3 days
Difficulty: Moderate
Recommended Maps and Other Resources:
- Monongahela National Forest, *Dolly Sods*, 2010
  www.fs.usda.gov/Internet/FSE_DOCUMENTS/stelprdb5152038.pdf.
- USGS Quads: Blackbird Knob, Hopeville, Blackwater Falls, and Laneville.

Dolly Sods's tundra-like environment of heaths, meadows, and scattered copses of red spruce is unlike any other in the Mid-Atlantic. Many observers remark that the landscape suggests Canada or even Alaska. Plan your visit for early summer or late autumn and you're likely to be treated to a riot of spring or fall color.

HIKE OVERVIEW

By walking a northward loop from Dolly Sods's Red Creek Trailhead, you'll gain a keen appreciation for the uniqueness of this Wilderness as you leave behind fairly typical Mid-Atlantic scenery and reach the wide open vistas of the "sods," a local term for high-altitude meadows and heaths. Tour all the highlights of this distinctive landscape and complete a walk-around of the periphery of the wilderness before returning via Red Creek and the rocky promontory of Lion's Head.

Dolly Sods boasts a unique environment in the Mid-Atlantic, and it also can throw some extreme weather your way. Snowfall can reach 150 inches a year, and winds have been recorded at 100 MPH. Before visiting, keep in mind that you can expect almost any form of weather, any time of the year; if bad weather finds you in the northern expanse of the Sods, you'll be exposed to the brunt of it. Time your visit for June through October, as the cooler weather on the plateau will be a welcome relief from the sweltering Mid-Atlantic summer.

HOW TO REACH THE TRAILHEAD

From the intersection of I-66 and I-81, take I-81 south toward Strasburg, Virginia. Leave the interstate at Exit 296 and head west on US 48/VA 55, which will become WV 55 when it crosses the border. Follow WV 55 about 43 miles to Moorefield, West Virginia, then turn left on US 220/WV 28. After about 13 miles, arrive in Petersburg, West Virginia; turn right on WV 28. About 10 miles outside of town, take a hard right onto CR 28/Jordan Run Road. At this point, the road becomes gravel, but it is well maintained and suitable for cars, when dry. Continue onto Forest Road 19, which will take you to the Red Creek trailhead, on the right, in about 10 miles (38° 58.371' N, 79° 23.8571' W).

About 4 miles from the trailhead, you'll pass Forest Road 75 on the right. This road is the easternmost boundary of the Wilderness and allows access to a number of additional trailheads (see Other Options).

Check on the status of these forest roads before heading out, as they can sometimes be affected by inclement weather; they can also still be closed late into spring. It is also possible to reach the trailhead from the west, using WV 32. This route may be longer, but the road is paved the entire way.

OVERNIGHT OPTIONS

Dolly Sods abounds in excellent backcountry camping, but given the popularity of some of these sites, stake your claim early. Limit the size of your group to ten people. If you bring dogs, they must be under their owners' control at all times.

Dunkenbarger Trail (4.1/3,683/39° 0.057' N, 79° 23.191' W). As you reach the edge of the plateau, the trail crosses a small run, where there is flat ground and a few established campsites.

Big Stonecoal (5.2/3,640/39° 0.317' N, 79° 22.574' W). Just as Dunkenbarger Trail intersects Big Stonecoal Trail, there are campsites with easy access to water. A few hundred yards north on Big Stonecoal, the trail crosses the creek; if you stay on the west bank, you'll quickly come upon a few additional sites.

Bear Rocks Trail (14.0/3,801/39° 03.849' N, 79° 19.388' W). Before this trail intersects with Dobbin Grade, it will dip down to Red Creek, cross it, and arrive at this campsite along the creek.

The Forks (18.6/3,492/39° 01.168' N, 79° 21.148' W). Clustered around the forks of Red Creek are the "must-have" campsites for this trip. With picturesque waterfalls and swimming holes nearby, this spot is deservedly sought after. Arrive early for the best sites.

Red Creek In its lower reaches, Red Creek Trail is dotted with tent sites, especially at trail intersections. Look for tent sites where Big and Little Stone-

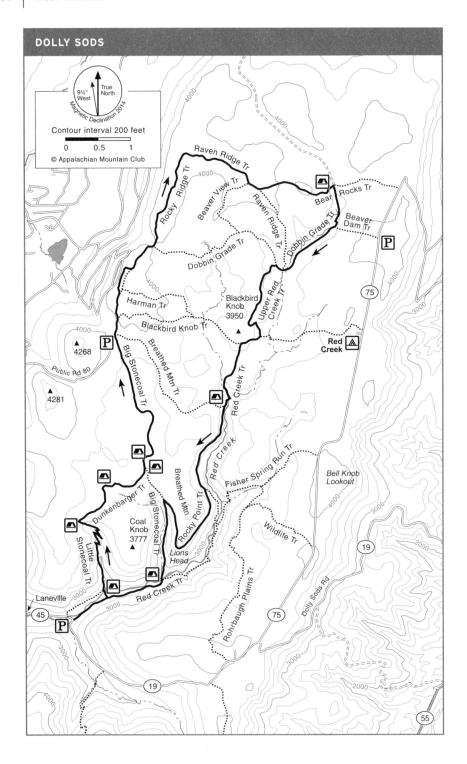

DOLLY SODS

coal Trails cross the river (23.1/2,801/38° 58.831' N, 79° 22.371' W) and (24/2,690/38° 58.709' N, 79° 23.320' W).

HIKE DESCRIPTION

For the entirety of the trip, keep your eyes peeled: the trails in the Dolly Sods Wilderness are not blazed. Intersections are signed fairly well, especially in the north, and there are cairns to help. You'll need to take heed to stay on trail, especially when crossing open areas.

From the trailhead's parking lot, begin walking east on Red Creek Trail (TR 514). At first, the treadway is big and broad and travels through typical Mid-Atlantic scenery, but it won't be long before the path rides up on the canyon wall to the right or crosses the occasional stream.

Soon, Red Creek's river bed widens out and arrives at a sign marking the crossing for Little Stonecoal Trail (TR 552; 0.6/2,685), which you'll follow northward into the Wilderness. Take care crossing the creek; it drains a significant expanse of terrain, and if it's swollen with rain or snowmelt, it could become dangerous.

(If Red Creek is too high to cross, there is a high water route on the north side of the creek. Cross on the bridge near the trailhead, then walk east along the north side of the creek along an old road grade. The trail peters out just shy of Little Stonecoal Trail, but you can bushwhack fairly easily along the river bank to find the trail. You could also follow Red Creek Trail farther into the Wilderness and hope for easier crossings higher up.)

The most substantial climb along this route, Little Stonecoal Trail climbs about a thousand feet over the next couple of miles, keeping always to the eastern side of the run. When the trail turns sharply to the east (right), a sign marks the trail's continuation as Dunkenbarger Trail (TR 558; 3.2/3,657). Keep an eye out for the cairns here, as the path can be hard to make out. Soon the path levels out through close forests of evergreens, jumps over a small tributary feeding Red Creek, and intersects with Big Stonecoal Trail (TR 513) (5.2/3,640). Bear straight onto this trail.

For the next 3 miles, walk northward along Big Stonecoal Trail. Initially, the trail follows the west side of the run, but it soon crosses (5.2/3,640). Watch for the cairns, as it's easy to walk by this ford. The path is fairly level, but it eventually weaves in and out of stands of trees, crossing open meadows where the path can become more difficult to discern. If in doubt, try to snoop out the trail along the forest edge. By the time you reach the intersection with Breathed Mountain Trail (TR 553) and Blackbird Knob Trail (TR 511), the forests will have largely yielded to the open heath for which the northern section of Dolly Sods is famed (7.96/3,920).

From this signed intersection, head north on Blackbird Knob Trail (TR 511), which branches eastward (8.2/4,006). Continue north on Rocky Ridge Trail (TR 524), walking over rolling tundra that offer increasingly big views of Canaan Valley in the west. Keep your eye out for Valley View Trail, a side trail on the left that will take you to the edge of the plateau and offer you access to a few rocky vantage points (8.57/4,130). Rejoin Rocky Ridge Trail after 1.16 miles (9.26/4,155) and continue north. Once you pass the intersection with Dobbin Grade Trail (9.73/3,996), you have some of the best walking in the Wilderness. The trail meanders around increasingly fantastic rock formations, many of which offer tantalizing outlooks of the surrounding highlands.

Rocky Ridge Trail and Raven Ridge Trail (TR 521) meet at the northwest corner of the Wilderness (11.4/4,155). Turn right on Raven Ridge Trail and begin walking eastward. The trail weaves its way into stands of red spruce, then follows the rolling, open terrain. Pass an intersection with Beaver View Trail (TR 523) on your right (12.5/4,108), and veer left at the next intersection onto Bear Rocks Trail (TR 522) (12.7/4,074). This trail descends rather sharply, crosses Red Creek, and finally reaches its intersection with Dobbin Grade Trail (TR 526; 14/3,819).

Over the next 2 miles, hike southward along boggy Dobbin Grade Trail. The grade itself is often exceptionally muddy. Even using the side trails that attempt to avoid the worst of the quicksand, you can find yourself up to your knees in mud on occasion. In spring or after a heavy rain, exercise caution when walking through this area. The trail crosses Red Creek (15.7/3,707) and passes the southern terminus of Raven Ridge Trail on the right. Head south (left) on Upper Red Creek Trail (TR 509; 15.9/3,712), which also crosses another tributary. Don't fret: your feet may well already be wet from crossing the grade.

Upper Red Creek Trail climbs away from the creek and approaches Blackbird Knob, rounding it on the east. On the eastern flank of this knob, take a right on Blackbird Knob Trail (TR 511; 17.3/3,765). Walk about a quarter-mile to the junction with Red Creek Trail (TR 514; 17.7/3,842), then head south (left). Red Creek Trail descends sharply away from the high heaths and bogs and into Mid-Atlantic forests until it reaches the Forks—an area where a number of prongs of Red Creek come together (18.6/3,489).

The trail wanders through lovely campsites, crosses one of the prongs across from a waterfall, and then rejoins a road grade on the right above the creek. If it helps, remember that you should leave the Forks walking downstream. The

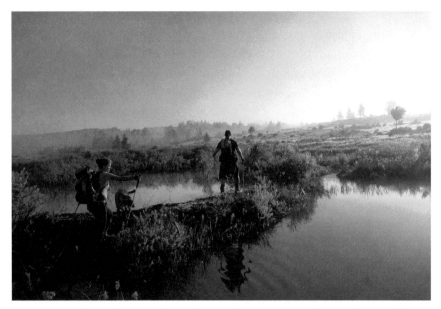

Backpackers thread their way through one of the many bogs that dot Dolly Sods's high tundra-like environment.

next stretch of Red Creek Trail sticks to this road grade, increasingly high on the right above Red Creek. Pass the intersection for the southern terminus of Breathed Mountain Trail (TR 553; 18.7/3,509), and turn right on Rocky Point Trail (TR 554; 20.1/3,314).

Bear right and follow this trail. The treadway becomes rocky and fractured as it rounds the point of Lion's Head (21.2/3,544). Scramble up the boulder fields for a view of Red Creek's drainage. Continue along Rocky Point Trail as it heads north and then intersects with the southern tail of Big Stonecoal Trail (21.9/3,566). Turn south (left) here and begin the quick, direct, and rather steep descent down to cross Red Creek one final time (23.1/2,806).

With the creek behind you, take a right on Red Creek Trail, and follow it to the trailhead, where your vehicle awaits (24.6/2,627). Though this last stretch of trail is not tame (it swings up onto the side of the canyon walls and sometimes proves difficult to find), you walked it on the way in, so it should not trouble you.

OTHER OPTIONS

If you prefer to do a shorter hike, enter the Wilderness using one of the trailheads along Forest Road 75 (Blackbird Knob Trailhead, Beaver Dam Trailhead, or Bear Rocks Trailhead). From these points, you'll be able to intercept this route via spur trails. You can easily walk a loop of 10–15 miles that will take you through all of the area's distinctive scenery, most of which is concentrated in the northern half of the Wilderness.

If you're looking to add miles, investigate the many trails that crisscross the Wilderness rather than staying on the periphery. Dolly Sods rewards exploration, and by base camping for a few nights and wandering about during the day, a backpacker could enjoy the Sods to the fullest. It's hard to imagine a more beautiful campsite than the Forks for this sort of expedition.

NEARBY

Petersburg and Seneca Rocks—and the road between the two settlements—are lined with businesses serving the hunters, climbers, skiers, hikers, backpackers, and other outdoorspeople who visit this area. You'll have no difficulty locating whatever service you need.

ADDITIONAL INFORMATION

To contact the Cheat-Potomac Ranger District, call 304-257-4488, ext. 0, or visit fs.usda.gov/recarea/mnf/recarea/?recid=12366.

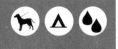

TRIP 9
WILD, WONDERFUL . . . AND WET:
OTTER CREEK

Location: Monongahela National Forest, West Virginia
Highlights: Hike along the pools, waterfalls, and cascades of a pristine creek deep in West Virginia's Otter Creek Wilderness
Distance: 16 miles round-trip
Total Elevation Gain/Loss: 3,314 feet gain/3,314 feet loss
Trip Length: 2–3 days
Difficulty: Moderate
Recommended Maps and Other Resources:
- Allen de Hart and Bruce Sundquist. *Monongahela National Forest Hiking Guide*, 8th ed. Charleston, WV: West Virginia Highlands Conservancy, 2006.
- USGS Quads: Parsons, Mozark Mountain, Bowden, and Harman.

Winding through its pristine Wilderness, Otter Creek is an enchanting walk at any time of year. With its cascading waterfalls, inviting swimming holes, and hidden vistas, you're more likely to find yourself sunning on the rocks than pushing hard into the evening. Early in the morning or at twilight, the sunlight dappling the river is a magical and memorable sight.

HIKE OVERVIEW

Officially designated as a Wilderness area in 1975, Otter Creek offers more of a backcountry experience than many lands within national forests or the National Park system, especially before and after summer crowds. Expect to find few blazes and fewer signs. The trails are meant to be accessible only to foot traffic, and not all of the deadfalls are removed as part of the maintenance that occurs. The Forest Service maintains the Wilderness this way to keep it wild, and it has done so successfully: the Wilderness is also one of the few areas in West Virginia where there is a healthy population of black bears.

In any season, the pools, rapids, eddies, and waterfalls of Otter Creek make for an extraordinary hike, particularly if you can time your visit so that there's ample water in the creek, but not so much that the four fords becomes excessively difficult. This is an excellent trip for setting up camp at a beautiful spot beside a swimming hole and doing some day-hiking along the tributary valleys. You could easily enjoy two or three nights of "slackpacking." You'll accomplish almost all of your hard climbing in the first 2 miles of the trail, and the only challenging descent comes as you follow Green Mountain Trail to Otter Creek. Otherwise the terrain is very moderate.

Crossing the four fords in this trip shouldn't be difficult much of the year, though you will likely get wet below the knees. If the water is higher, however, consider whether the creek is crossable. Rushing water is potentially quite dangerous, and you don't want to be out in the middle of a river and realize that you have miscalculated and the stream is stronger than you. If you plan on visiting in spring when Otter Creek could be swollen with snowmelt, call the ranger station in advance to inquire. In any season, be wise and reroute your trip if necessary. You might have to settle for seeing the Wilderness only on one side of the creek.

A firm word of caution: remember that there are no signs to speak of in the Otter Creek Wilderness and any blazes that remain are fading quickly. Route-finding is not especially difficult, but you do need to keep a careful eye out for the trail in spots. Beginners should be especially aware and prepared.

OVERNIGHT OPTIONS

Backcountry camping is allowed throughout the forest, without a permit, but keep your party size small (under ten) and always follow Leave No Trace procedures. Camping is not permitted near trailheads or trail intersections, and you should gather only dead wood for campfires. Use of stoves for cooking is strongly encouraged. Carry out, or burn, used toilet paper.

Shavers Mountain Trail (3.92/3,723/38° 59.575' N, 79° 36.217' W). If you start in late afternoon or early evening, you may want to camp near the four-way intersection marked by a cairn. Turning left or right will take you, in short order, to a few backcountry sites with fire rings. There is a rumor of a spring on the left, but I could not find it in October. It is likely seasonal, so if you plan to camp here, you'd do best to treat it as a dry camp.

Possession Camp Trail (5.7/3,422/39° 0.578' N, 79° 36.991' W). If you have the daylight, head to this campsite at the intersection of Green Mountain Trail and Possession Camp Trail. There's a spring nearby.

Lower Otter Creek (8.63/2,236/39° 1.358' N, 79° 39.108' W). These campsites are on the left, just after you turn onto Otter Creek Trail from Green Mountain Trail. A particularly nice campsite is on the right after the first ford (8.9/2,240/39° 1.259' N, 79° 39.029' W).

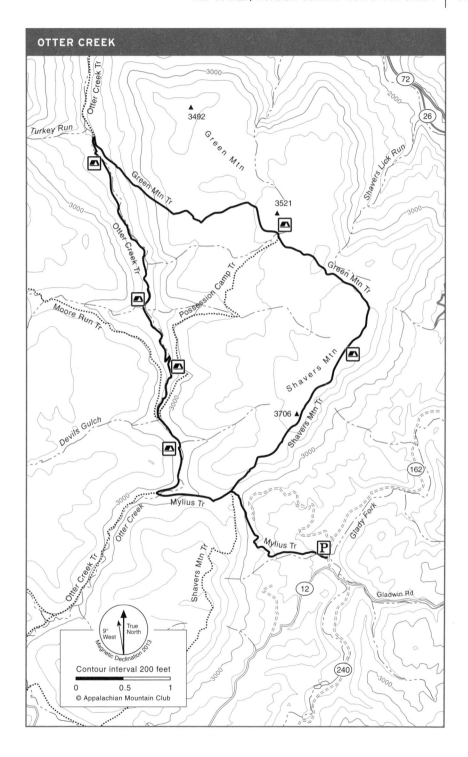

Moore's Run (10.6/2,537/38° 59.985' N, 79° 38.577' W). Just after the trail crosses Moore's Run, an uphill path leads to a lovely campsite within easy reach of several wonderful swimming holes.

Upper Otter Creek (starting at 12/2,709/38° 59.339' N, 79° 38.272' W). Between the second and third fords of Otter Creek, there are a number of excellent camping sites, with plenty of space for several tents. One has a few built-up stone benches, but it is located right on the trail.

HOW TO REACH THE TRAILHEAD

From I-81, take Exit 296 and head west on US 48/VA 55. After you enter West Virginia, continue to Moorefield on WV 55. In Moorefield, turn left onto WV 28 and follow it through Petersburg and on to Seneca Rocks. There, bear right onto US 33 and drive about 22.6 miles. Turn right onto CR 12/Sully Road. This turnoff is marked by the Alpine Lodge and Restaurant, so you can't miss it. Proceed about 4.5 miles along CR 12 almost to a bridge. Take a hard left onto FR 162. The parking lot for Mylius Trail is just a few hundred feet up the road on the left (38° 57.706' N, 79° 36.469' W).

HIKE DESCRIPTION

From the trailhead, Mylius Trail begins ascending a gentle road grade for a few hundred yards. The path is blazed blue, but don't get too used to those blazes—they won't be there for long. The trail veers to the left away from the road, crosses a power cut and a clearing, and then gets a little more serious about climbing. As you approach a barbed wire fence on the left, the road grade turns sharply to the right, as if it intends to switchback up the mountain (0.6/2,630). Don't follow it; instead, look for the footpath that follows the barbed wire fence for a few hundred feet. That's your trail. (If, by some mischance, you miss the footpath, you won't go far. The little road is obstructed by blowdowns and comes to an end entirely in just a few tenths of a mile.)

Eventually, the trail leaves the fence, climbs steeply for a bit, and then settles into a comfortable, rightward traversing climb that dips through a few hollows on its way to the intersection with Shavers Mountain Trail. Mylius Trail eventually arrives at a broad saddle on the shoulder of the mountain where two trails come together (1.65/3,171). This is the intersection with Shavers Mountain Trail; you've climbed about 900 feet of the total 1,300 feet. There is a fire pit here, but camping is prohibited (a legal campsite is farther ahead).

Turn right on Shavers Mountain Trail. After 400 more feet of climbing, the path reaches the top of Shavers Mountain and spends several level miles crossing the broad top of this ridge, with partially obscured views of the Alleghenies to

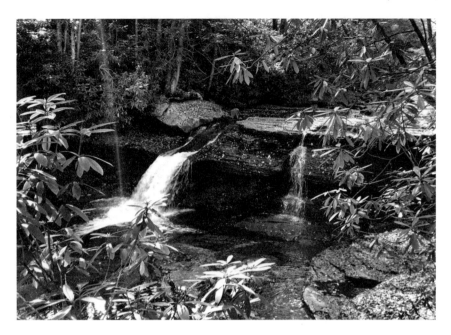

If you time your visit right, the waterworks of Otter Creek offer some of the best swimming holes in the region.

the right. At times, the trail takes you through stands of evergreens that loom close over the path; at other times, it opens out into broader areas. After almost 2 miles of walking (3.92/3,723), you'll reach a four-way intersection. The path ahead of you is marked by a cairn; the other paths are unmarked. Turn left or right to reach the Shavers Mountain Trail campsites.

When you're ready to proceed, continue straight. Just about 0.5 mile beyond this point (4.5/3,602), the trail descends slightly to a "Trail Abandoned" sign. Find Green Mountain Trail to the left. This trail winds through forests of rhododendron on its way to Otter Creek and, in early spring, it must be quite a sight. At times, however, the footing can be rather boggy. After about 1.25 miles, Green Mountain Trail reaches the turnoff for Possession Camp Trail on the left and a campsite and spring at the intersection (5.7/3,422).

Stay on Green Mountain Trail to the right and continue along some broad and relatively open avenues between the trees. Just before it begins its descent, Green Mountain Trail turns sharply right (7.2/3,298). From there, the trail heads directly down the mountains and at times grows steep, rocky, and brambly as it plunges about 1,000 feet into the Otter Creek hollow.

At the bottom of its descent, Green Mountain Trail bumps into Otter Creek Trail (8.4/2,205). Take a sharp turn leftward on Otter Creek Trail to reach the campsites of the lower creek in about 0.25 mile. Just beyond the first couple of campsites, the trail also turns sharply right and introduces you to your first ford of Otter Creek, which is marked on both banks by cairns (8.86/2,239).

When it comes to the technique of crossing a ford, there are different schools of thought. There are the rock-hoppers, the shoe-removers, and the wet-feet-walkers. I won't engage in a lengthy polemic about what is best, since passions run high. I believe, however, that all of these groups will agree that trekking poles are a serious help when crossing Otter Creek's fords, especially as the algae-covered rocks can be slippery.

Once you cross the first ford, the trail follows the right bank of the river for much of the length of this section of Otter Creek. At times, the trail grows narrow and rides up high over the creek; at other moments, the trail dips down low beside the creek and follows former road grades. These sections feel almost like tree-lined avenues. Take your time. When the opportunity arises, take the side trails to the creek bed—there are many picturesque views of the waterworks that you'll enjoy. When I walked the trail, there was one section along the creek so badly eroded that it could not be followed. Just walk down to the creek bed, follow it for a few feet and rejoin the trail on the other side.

After about 2 miles, Otter Creek Trail reaches the little rocky shelves that signal the confluence of Moore's Run (10.6/2,537). A small trail leads up Moore's Run to the right, but to follow Otter Creek, cross the run and head up the far bank. The next section of the trail is perhaps the most beautiful. After passing the gorgeous campsite to the right, the trail offers a few sections where you can reach the water to obtain views of swimming holes and waterfalls. Several large rocks invite sunbathing or general loafing.

Otter Creek Trail then reaches the second ford (12.0/2,701), crosses to the left side of the creek, and passes a number of campsites, all of good quality, though several are very close to the trail. The third ford comes hard on the heels of the second (12.9/2,869), with a broad campsite just past it. If you're walking on, note that the trail turns hard left after the crossing; you don't need to enter the campsite to find it.

The remaining stretch of Otter Creek trail is less striking. The trail follows an old road grade and veers away from the creek bed on the right. Soon the trail reaches a three-way intersection with Yellow Creek Trail, which continues on straight. Turn left, ford Otter Creek a fourth and final time, and begin ascending along Mylius Trail (13.6/2,909), which is big and broad, though a bit boggy in spots. The trail crosses a small creek, and then becomes more of a footpath. After approximately 300 feet of gentle climbing, it arrives at the intersection of Shavers Mountain Trail (14.3/3,171). You turned north here when you walked in from the car. To return to the trailhead (16.0/2,318), go straight and retrace your steps as you descend the rightward traversing trail.

OTHER OPTIONS

If you are looking for more trails to hike, you have more than a few choices, but keep these in mind:

- Yellow Creek Trail and Moore Run Trail offer tempting opportunities for day-hiking or for finding a more secluded spot off the beaten path. Both trails follow tributaries to Otter Creek.
- Big Springs Gap is a more northerly trailhead accessing Otter Creek. Enter the Wilderness from here and avoid the up-and-over approach via Shavers Mountain and Green Mountain trails. Other trailheads exist to the west and south of Otter Creek along Forest Roads 91 and 324.
- Ascend Mylius Trail, bypass the right-hand turn on Shavers Mountain Trail, and continue straight to where Yellow Creek Trail and Otter Creek intersect. This approach will get you to the campsites along upper Otter Creek much faster, but you'll lose the charm of walking up the creek bed.

NEARBY

As you approach Seneca Rocks, West Virginia, you'll be entering a sportsperson's paradise that caters to outdoorspeople of all different stripes. You won't have any difficulty finding a room for the night, if you desire. Seneca Rocks is a mecca for rock climbers on the East Coast, so stop in for last-minute camping supplies or to replace a forgotten piece of gear.

ADDITIONAL INFORMATION

For more information, contact the Cheat Ranger District, Monongahela National Forest, Elkins, West Virginia, at 304-636-1800.

TRIP 10
(DON'T) GET LOST!

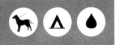

Location: Monongahela National Forest, West Virginia

Highlights: Immaculate solitude, gorgeous views from the Canyon Rim Trail, route-finding challenges, and the picturesque South Prong of Red Creek

Distance: 13.4 miles round-trip

Total Elevation Gain/Loss: 2,587 feet gain/2,587 feet loss

Trip Length: 2–3 days

Difficulty: Challenging

Recommended Maps and Other Resources:

- Michael V. Juskelis. *The Mid-Atlantic Hiker's Guide: West Virginia: Sixty-four Day Hikes and Weekend Backpacking Trips for Novices and Experts.* Spring Mills, PA: Scott Adams Enterprises, 2013.
- Allen de Hart and Bruce Sundquist. *Monongahela National Forest Hiking Guide,* 8th ed. Charleston, WV: West Virginia Highlands Conservancy, 2006.
- USGS Quads: Laneville and Hopeville.

High above the eastern seaboard, West Virginia's Roaring Plains offer you view after view of the mountainous horizon as you follow cairns along the rugged and rocky canyon rim. An ideal summer trip; consider timing your visit for late July or early August when the trails are aisles amid the blueberry bushes.

HIKE OVERVIEW

From the trailhead on Forest Road 19, this route will take you up Boars Nest Trail to the Flatrock Plains and Roaring Plains—at 4,000 feet, this plateau is among the highest in the Eastern United States. Among red spruce, open brushy terrain, and bogs, you'll feel you've reached a completely different environment as you take in nearly endless views of the Alleghenies along Canyon Rim Trail and the Hidden Passage.

If you enjoy a good route-finding challenge, then this trip is certainly for you. While the hiking is not especially strenuous, keeping on these trails is as tough as anything in this book. Though the area is fairly small and bound by several well-defined features, it is quite possible to get turned around. Nearly impenetrable thickets of mountain laurel and rhododendron make bushwhacking in a straight line exceedingly difficult, if not impossible. This trip is not intended for the novice route-finder. You should have a map, a compass, and a GPS unit with you, and you should know how to use them. Also, follow good hiking safety protocol—bring a buddy and make sure you tell a friend or loved one of your plans.

HOW TO REACH THE TRAILHEAD

From the intersection of I-81 and I-66, head south on I-81 to Exit 296. Take a right and head west on US 48/VA 55. In West Virginia, this road will become a broad, four-lane highway. After about 43 miles, take the exit for Moorefield, West Virginia. In town, hang a left on US 220 and follow it about 13 miles to Petersburg. There, take a right on WV 28. Ten miles later, take a sharp right onto Jordan Run Road. Turn left on Forest Road 19/Dolly Sods Road in about 1 mile. Follow this gravel road into the mountains. Near the Dolly Sods Picnic Area, you'll pass a trailhead on the left for South Prong Trail, which ends here. Continue down Forest Road 19. You'll lose elevation and eventually come to the trailhead for Boars Nest Trail and the other end of South Prong Trail. Park here (38° 57.6769' N, 79° 23.3535' W).

OVERNIGHT OPTIONS

Backcountry camping is permitted, without a permit, in Roaring Plains and Flatrock Plains. You'll have several excellent spots to choose from.

Upper South Fork of Red Creek (2.45/4,157/38° 55.990' N, 79° 23.503' W). Just after you complete the climb to the high country, the trail leads you into a wooded copse where Boars Nest Trail crosses the creek. This is a beautiful spot with plenty of tent sites and water.

North Canyon Rim Trail (4.47/4,598/38° 55.181' N, 79° 24.613' W). You may be in the mood for a rest after completing Tee Pee Trail. If so, consider this campsite at the intersection with Canyon Rim Trail. It has easy access to several fantastic views, but you'll need to carry in your own water.

South Canyon Rim Trail (5.76/4,342/38° 54.570' N, 79° 23.697' W). A similar site is available farther south on Canyon Rim Trail, just shy of where the trail takes a northward turn. Again, there's easy access to views, but no water without hiking for it.

Hidden Passage (8.5/4,440/38° 55.252' N, 79° 22.494' W). There are two excellent campsites along this trail: the first is dry but is located near wide open views of the eastern mountains, the second is located on a branch flowing into the South Prong (9.89/4,093/38° 55.976' N, 79° 21.962' W).

ROARING PLAINS

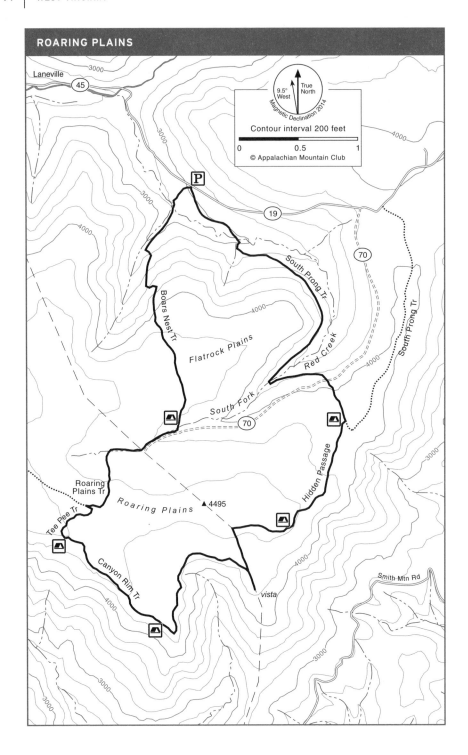

Contour interval 200 feet

0   0.5   1

© Appalachian Mountain Club

HIKE DESCRIPTION

At the trailhead, orient yourself: the forest road leading southeast is South Prong Trail, the path on which you'll be returning. Locate Boars Nest Trail by walking to the road and looking left to find the southwest-bound footpath headed downhill. You can spot several blue plastic tags on the trees.

Boars Nest Trail begins by descending about 200 feet to the South Prong of Red Creek (0.3/2,796). Although this crossing may not be especially difficult in drier times, be cautious if there's recently been a great deal of rain or snowmelt. On the far bank, the trail begins a stout climb of about 1,500 feet over the next 1.73 miles, first following a little creek, and then leaving it to switchback up the mountain. As you top out this climb (2.0/4,290), you'll immediately sense the unique environment of Flatrock Plains and Roaring Plains, with their thickets of brush and expansive bogs. Turn back to get a view of Dolly Sods behind you, then walk on to the upper reaches of South Prong (2.45/4,157), which you can easily rock hop. If you're planning to camp at a dry site farther along, fill your bottles here.

Take a right on Forest Road 70 (2.53/4,159) and walk along it for just 0.4 mile before you reach a pipeline cut (2.89/4,229). Look across it, slightly to the right, and you'll spot Roaring Plains Trail, which you should follow for another 0.9 mile of easy walking (3.8/4,512).

And now for the navigational crux of this trip—finding Tee Pee Trail. At almost 1 mile on Roaring Plains Trail, you should spot a cairn marking a left turn onto a path (38° 55.413' N, 79° 24.396' W). Take that turn, and then very soon afterwards take a right onto a fainter trail (3.9/4,504/ 38° 55.393' N, 79° 24.345' W). At that point, you should be on a southwestward bearing. Do not continue to walk southeast on the first path, as that will take you to the eastern end of Canyon Rim Trail. Tee Pee Trail can be quite rugged and obscured by blowdowns, but it basically follows a southwestward bearing to the campsite marking the beginning of the Canyon Rim Trail (4.47/4,598/38° 55.181' N, 79° 24.613' W). Entering these coordinates into your GPS device before the trip will make navigating this particular zig-zag much more feasible.

Once you've reached Canyon Rim Trail, navigating becomes easier, though you won't be able to go completely on automatic. Marked by cairns, this occasionally very rocky trail follows the rim southeast for 1.5 miles, bringing you to a series of rocky outcroppings offering dramatic views and excellent opportunities for photographs. Enjoy these places, but be careful as well. Rattlesnakes love to sun themselves on these dry shelves.

After passing these gorgeous views, the trail turns north (5.9/4,321) and follows the rim to a small creek (6.5/4,233). You may be rather dry by now,

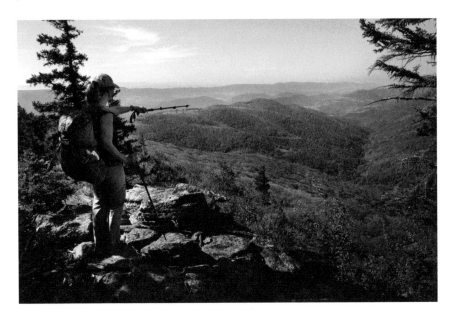

Canyon Rim Trail features breathtaking vistas of West Virginia's Allegheny highlands.

so it's a good idea to get water. Past this creek, the trail bends around to the east, veers away from the rim, and traverses a forested area before reaching the pipeline cut (7.2/4,253). A short walk down the cut will take you to a good viewpoint (7.43/4,268).

Heading north, the pipeline cut climbs for about 0.3 mile from where the trail originally reached it. Look to the right at the top of the rise, and you'll see a grassy old jeep trail (8.0/4,459). This is the fabled Hidden Passage (38° 55.231' N, 79° 23.019' W), which has seen enough traffic that it is no longer so hidden. Take the right, and follow Hidden Passage through an open area, with big views of the Alleghenies to the east. Eventually, the path comes to a campsite in a wooded area; here the trail becomes more of a footpath (8.47/4,443). You may have to fumble around a bit to find Hidden Passage, but it generally continues northeastward and starts to descend slightly.

After almost 1.5 miles of walking, the trail reaches a campsite on your left (9.89/4,093) and crosses the creek to your right. Here, Hidden Passage joins South Prong Trail (10/4,100); you should be able to spot blue plastic blazes. Bear left, and begin the gradual descent to your vehicle.

South Prong Trail crosses Forest Road 70 (10.4/3,887), and then descends into the hollow where Red Creek flows. After the path crosses the creek (11/3,734), it follows an old road grade as it rounds the foot of the mountain. A steeper descent brings you down to Red Creek (12.8/2,974). With one more crossing behind you, walk a gently ascending, grassy forest road until you find your vehicle (13.4/3,018).

OTHER OPTIONS

If you'd like to make this trip significantly easier, park at the upper trailhead for South Prong Trail and walk in to Hidden Passage, thus avoiding the climb up Boars Nest Trail. Walking the trail counterclockwise also has the advantage of simplifying your task in locating Tee Pee Trail; if you're not using a GPS, or not entirely confident as a route-finder, you should consider walking the trip in reverse.

If you're thinking you'd like to add miles, Roaring Plains Trail will take you into the western portion of the Wilderness. Additionally, Rohrbaugh Trail (with a trailhead on the right as you drive west on FR 19) would allow you access to Dolly Sods (Trip 8) and link together a longer exploration of this beautiful area.

NEARBY

Moorefield and Petersburg, West Virginia, are the nearest towns; they offer a good array of businesses, many of which cater to the tourists and outdoorspeople exploring wild and wonderful West Virginia.

ADDITIONAL INFORMATION

For additional information, visit the Monongahela National Forest's website at fs.usda.gov/mnf or contact the Cheat-Potomac Ranger District at 304-257-4488, ext. 0.

TRIP 11
CARRYING WATER

Location: Monongahela National Forest, West Virginia
Highlights: Views of the most rugged mountains in West Virginia, Chimney Top
Distance: 23.5 miles one-way
Total Elevation Gain/Loss: 3,839 feet gain/6,297 feet loss
Trip Length: 2–3 days
Difficulty: Challenging
Recommended Maps and Other Resources:

- Allen de Hart and Bruce Sundquist. *Monongahela National Forest Hiking Guide*, 8th ed. Charleston, WV: West Virginia Highlands Conservancy, 2006. The best available maps ship with this book.
- USGS Quads: Petersburg West, Hopeville, and Upper Tract.

If you study a topographic map of West Virginia's most popular hiking regions, you're bound to notice North Fork Mountain's long, straight ridgeline driving like a dagger through many of the region's highlights, including Seneca Rocks, Spruce Knob, Dolly Sods, and Roaring Plains. It's even harder to miss North Fork Mountain's impressive sandstone cliffs in person. For many backpackers in the region, completing 23.5-mile North Fork Mountain Trail is a bucket-list must—despite the demanding challenges it presents.

HIKE OVERVIEW

This northbound end-to-end trip offers impressive vistas and rugged miles, and climaxes with rock scrambling on Chimney Top and then a quick descent to the valley floor. By starting in the south, you'll keep the amount of climbing to be done relatively low.

Give serious consideration to your water needs as you plan. If you intend to hike the trail swiftly, you may be able to carry your own water for the entire trip. If you're planning to go slower or linger up high, consider caching water at the midpoint of the trail, along Forest Road 79. Doing so will make the trip's logistics more complicated, but your load will be lighter. How much water should you carry? The answer depends on you and your needs, so it's best to observe how much water you ordinarily use and carry a little extra. In my case, in July, I carried 6 liters and used it all. If you should get in a bind regarding water, remember that all of the eastward-leading trails and roads will eventually take you to water.

HOW TO REACH THE TRAILHEAD

To Reach the Ending Trailhead. From the intersection of I-66 and I-81, drive about 4 miles south on I-81, then take Exit 296 for US 48/VA 55. Follow this two-lane road west as it winds over the mountains on the border between Virginia and West Virginia and eventually reaches Wardensville, West Virginia. From there, WV 55 becomes a four-lane highway that brings you to Moorefield. Take a left on US 220/WV 28 and head south about 13 miles to the town of Petersburg. Take a right onto WV 28 and drive about 7 miles west. Then turn left on Smoke Hole Road. Cross the river and find the northern parking lot for North Fork Mountain Trail (38° 58.8908' N, 79° 13.871' W).

To Reach the Starting Trailhead. Return to WV 28 and take a left. Drive south about 26 miles, passing Seneca Rocks on the left. Then, bear left onto US 33. The road will climb to the top of North Fork Mountain. You'll know you've reached the top when you spot a radio antenna on the left. Park on the left shoulder (38° 42.6505' N, 79° 24.1222' W). The southern trailhead is past the gate, behind the antenna.

OVERNIGHT OPTIONS

Those willing to endure the passing discomfort of carrying or caching all their water will be treated to some excellent campsites with easy access to expansive views of the Alleghenies and Spruce Knob (West Virginia's highest point at 4,863).

Seneca Rocks Vista (8.05/3,660/38° 48.607' N, 79° 20.456' W). A cairn to the left of this summit—one of the trail's high points—marks a path leading to the best campsite on the southern half of the trail, which features ample room for tents. Beyond the remnants of an old gravel road, you can reach cliffs with a spectacular view of Seneca Rocks and Germany Valley, far below.

Mid Point (12.4/3,138/38° 51.682' N, 79° 18.726' W). After walking along Forest Road 79 for almost 2 miles, the trail heads straight while the road veers to the right. There is room for camping on the grassy margin to the left, but if you walk about 300 yards farther along (away from the road), another fair-sized (and more secluded) site sits on the broad back of the ridge. Caching water along Forest Road 79 is a wise plan.

Intersection of Redman Run (16/2,942/38° 54.349' N, 79° 16.822' W). This may not be the most interesting campsite along this route, but it is usefully

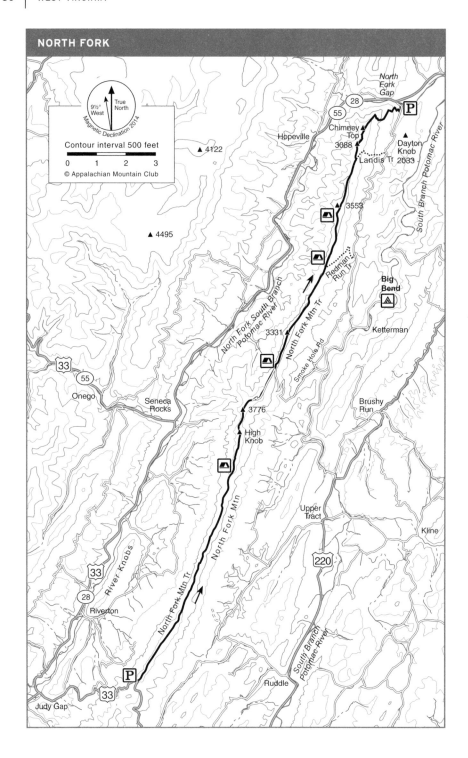

positioned. As you reach the intersection with Redman Run Trail, look to the right and you'll spot the fire ring.

North Point (18/3,399/38° 56.052' N, 79° 16.268' W). About halfway between the intersection for Redman Run Trail and Landis Trail, a good-sized campsite is located on the left. This is the best large site in the northern half of the trail.

A number of small campsites with easy access to views can be found around Chimney Top and on the descent from the ridgeline. These come late in the trip, but they could make excellent campsites if you were predisposed to linger an extra night.

HIKE DESCRIPTION

From the shoulder on top of the pass, begin your northbound thru-hike of North Fork Mountain Trail by passing the gate and walking north past the communications relay. Behind it, you'll come upon a fork in the trail. A jeep path bears leftward, while the blue-blazed trail bears right and passes between signs warning of private property. Be sure to stay on the trail! You'll generally find it broad and easy to follow, though there can be extended stretches between blazes.

Almost 8 miles of easy walking follow as the trail begins the trek north along the ridge's broad back. If you aren't pressed to cover miles, take the time to explore the side trails that lead to the ridgeline, as a number of them will bring you to beautiful views westward. After crossing a power cut (3.36/3,307), you'll spot a wooden platform higher up on the ridge to the left (4.49/3,362). Climb up to enjoy a beautiful view of Germany Valley and the North Fork of the South Branch of the Potomac River below. The ridge opposite includes Spruce Knob, West Virginia's highest point. Savor this vista, but be careful on the rocks. Rattlesnakes love to sun themselves here.

The trail undulates over the next 3.2 miles, and then climbs fairly steeply (7.77/3,488). Once you crest this climb, leave North Fork Mountain Trail to follow a short side path to the left. Marked by a cairn, this trail passes the Seneca Rocks Vista campsite and an impressive view of Seneca Rocks far below. After staying up high for the next 2.7 miles, North Fork Mountain Trail meets Forest Road 79 (10.2/3,764). Take a right on this road and follow the blue blazes, past a pipeline cut (10.6/3,783). Descend along the road, which twists and turns more than you would guess.

Eventually, it turns hard right and gets serious about descending the mountain, while North Fork Mountain Trail and your route continue along the ridgeline (12.2/3,088). (If you were going to cache water, this intersection would be

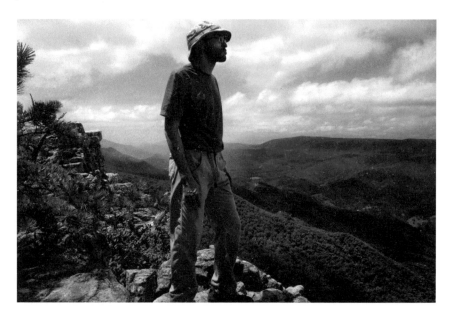

A backpacker surveys Germany Valley and Seneca Rocks from Chimney Top, high atop North Fork Mountain.

a good place to do it.) After it passes a campsite on the left (12.4/3,138), the trail follows the sloped east side of the mountain for several miles. Enjoy the views of the mountains, ranked like soldiers to the east, but keep your eye on the trail, as this is the least often walked section. Soon enough, North Fork Mountain Trail intersects with Redman Run Trail on the right (16/2,942).

Shortly after this intersection, the trail climbs, passing through tunnels of rhododendron, which are spectacular if they're blooming. Keep your eyes peeled for side trails opening up to outstanding views westward. When you reach the intersection with Landis Trail (20.0/2,852), be careful to bear left. North Fork Mountain Trail ascends about 200 feet more, and you should soon be able to catch a glimpse of the dramatic Chimney Top rock formation ahead of you (20.4/3,033). The trail to this beautiful feature is unmarked, however; remember to look out for it on the left (21/2,943). If you start to descend sharply, you've gone too far.

The spur trail to Chimney Top is steep and there are many branching trails, so you may have to persevere to reach the formation, but the views—of the Allegheny Front, Roaring Plains, and Dolly Sods to the west—are well worth it. It's impossible to get lost here, as you're hemmed in by the cliffs on the west and the Alleghenies on the east.

Once you've slaked your thirst with this amazing view, you may be ready refill your water bottles too, so it's time to descend from the ridgeline. With 1,900 feet to drop down to Smoke Hole Road, the descent is rocky and moderately steep in sections, but the trail winds around the northern edge of the ridgeline, offering you additional viewpoints of the valley below. Eventually, the descent eases off into a series of switchbacks and brings you to your vehicle and, best of all, the nearby North Fork of the South Branch of the Potomac (23.5/1,128). To complete the trip, you have only to reverse the shuttle.

OTHER OPTIONS

It's not practical to add mileage onto North Fork Mountain Trail, but there are several ways the trip could be shortened. Instead of starting at US 33, position the southernmost vehicle where Forest Road 79 meets the trail. Then, walk the northern half of the trail and, of course, visit Chimney Top. An even shorter route could be planned by continuing south on Smokehole Road after dropping off the first vehicle. Start the hike at the trailhead for Redman Run, climb to North Fork Mountain Trail, and then follow the last portion of the route as described.

Note that if you do decide to cache water or food along this route, Forest Road 79 is the key, as it will allow access to the trail's center point.

NEARBY

Seneca Rocks is a notable hangout for outdoorspeople of all stripes (especially climbers), and it offers a number of services. If you can't find what you're looking for there, keep a sharp eye out in Petersburg and Moorefield, West Virginia, as each features a range of businesses.

ADDITIONAL INFORMATION

For additional information about the North Fork Mountain Trail, contact the Monongahela National Forest at 304-636-1800.

TRIP 12
KING IN HIS CASTLE

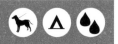

Location: George Washington and Jefferson National Forests, West Virginia

Highlights: Big Schloss, Tibbet Knob, Halfmoon Mountain, and the picturesque Trout Run

Distance: 27 miles round-trip

Total Elevation Gain/Loss: 5,479 feet gain/5,479 feet loss

Trip Length: 2–4 days

Difficulty: Moderate

Recommended Maps and Other Resources:

- Potomac Appalachian Trail Club, *Map F, Trails in Great North Mountain—North Half of George Washington National Forest, Lee Ranger District—Virginia and West Virginia.*
- Potomac Appalachian Trail Club, *Guide to Great North Mountain Trails.* Vienna, VA. Potomac Appalachian Trail Club, 2008.
- USGS Quads: Wolf Gap, Wardensville, Baker, and Woodstock.

Perched atop the dramatic sandstone cliffs of Big Schloss, you'll enjoy sweeping views of Trout Run Valley and the mountains guarding the border between Virginia and West Virginia. Named by German immigrants, Big Schloss means "big castle," and from this vantage point, you'll feel like a sovereign as you peer down at the route you've walked.

HIKE OVERVIEW

Circumnavigating Trout Run Valley is a worthy ambition for a beginner or intermediate backpacker looking to acquire skill and improve stamina. In agreeable weather, it's also a lovely walk with multiple lookout points, an abundance of attractive campsites, and terrain that varies from easy walking ground to short sections of scrambling. Start at Wolf Gap and walk south to the views along Tibbet Knob before proceeding north along Long Mountain. Past the idyllic Trout Run, climb Halfmoon Mountain for splendid views of the entire valley, then ridge walk south along Great North Mountain to Big Schloss, the highlight of the route.

HOW TO REACH THE TRAILHEAD

From the intersection of I-81 and I-66, drive south about 17 miles on I-81. Take Exit 283 for VA 42 near Woodstock, Virginia. Bear right onto VA 42, and head west about 5 miles. Take a right onto SR 768, which quickly merges with SR 623. Turn right onto SR 675/Wolf Gap Road. Climb along this increasingly mountainous road until it reaches the border of Virginia and West Virginia. After about 6 miles, you'll reach Wolf Gap. Turn right into the parking lot, where you can park your vehicle overnight (38° 55.4503' N, 78° 41.3647' W).

OVERNIGHT OPTIONS

You'll have no difficulty finding campsites on this loop. No backcountry permits are required, and campfires are allowed.

Tibbet Knob (1.71/2,930/38° 54.922' N, 78° 42.276' W). I mention this site in Trip 1. It's a gem, even if it is very near the start of this circuit. As you head south along yellow-blazed Tibbet Knob Trail, there are additional places to camp.

Long Mountain Trail (7.7/2,031/38° 57.852' N, 78° 43.172' W). Walking along yellow-blazed Long Mountain Trail, you'll spot a number of potential campsites, including several in clearings. The water situation can be questionable, however, as the runoff in this valley tends to be swallowed by sinkholes. The best campsites come as the trail descends to CR 23/20. Both before and after the bridge over Trout Run (13.1/1,434 and 13.6/1,455), you'll find attractive tenting sites with easy access to water.

Halfmoon Run (16.5/1,926/38° 59.717' N, 78° 38.225' W). As pink-blazed Bucktail Cut Off Trail winds its way through the hollows on the south face of Halfmoon Mountain, you'll spot a few backcountry sites. The best of these is a good-sized campsite where the trail intersects with the yellow-blazed Halfmoon Trail. You'll find plenty of water.

Halfmoon Lookout Trail (18.3/2,759/39° 0.033' N, 78° 37.892' W). If you have the urge to camp high and dry, there is a plum of a campsite waiting for you just a few vertical feet below the summit of Halfmoon Mountain. Just as the lookout trail turns uphill steeply, look to the left and you'll spot this small-ish campsite. Other, less scenic sites are in the saddle where yellow-blazed Halfmoon Trail intersects with white-blazed Halfmoon Lookout Trail.

Sandstone Spring (23.3/2,783/38° 57.328' N, 78° 39.253' W). While they don't offer the views of Halfmoon Mountain, the popular campsites at Sandstone Spring do have reliable water (the only water source on Mill Mountain Trail), and there are excellent views nearby.

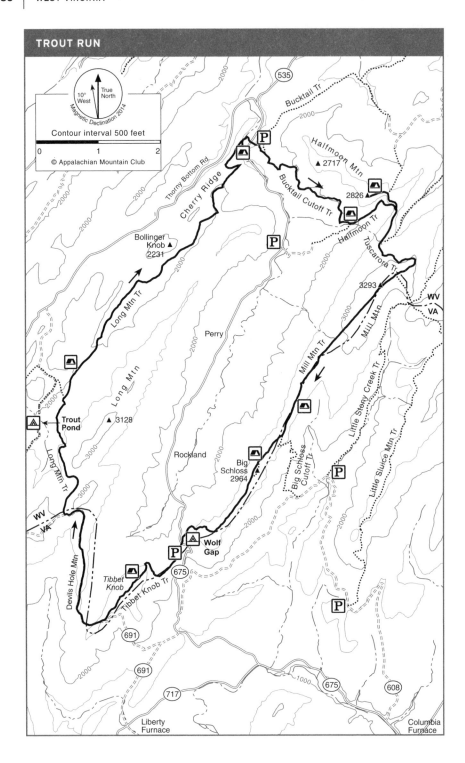

TROUT RUN

10° West / True North

Magnetic Declination 2014

Contour interval 500 feet

0   1   2

© Appalachian Mountain Club

535

Bucktail Tr

Halfmoon Mtn

▲ 2717

2826 ▲

Bucktail Cutoff Tr

Thorny Bottom Rd

Cherry Ridge

Bollinger Knob ▲ 2231

Halfmoon Tr

Tuscarora Tr

3293 ▲

WV
VA

Long Mtn Tr

Perry

Long Mtn

Mill Mtn

Mill Mtn Tr

▲ 3128

Trout Pond

Long Mtn Tr

Rockland

Big Schloss 2964

Big Schloss Cutoff Tr

Little Stony Creek Tr

Little Sluice Mtn Tr

P

WV
VA

Devils Hole Mtn

Wolf Gap

P

675

Tibbet Knob

Tibbet Knob Tr

691

691

717

Liberty Furnace

1000

675

608

Columbia Furnace

Big Schloss (24.5/2,964/38° 56.4832' N, 78° 39.9490' W). It may get crowded on top of this popular overlook, but there are a few narrow tent sites that certainly offer big views.

Established camping sites are at Wolf Gap and Trout Pond recreation areas.

HIKE DESCRIPTION

Walk south from Wolf Gap's parking lot and locate orange-blazed Tibbet Knob Trail. Over the next few hundred yards, the trail ascends gently to a ridgeline with views eastward to the Blue Ridge. It passes along the right shoulder of the ridge before climbing, steeply at times, toward the knob. Two sections require scrambling before you reach the views of Trout Run Valley from Tibbet Knob (1.5/2,926/38° 54.8560' N, 78° 42.2994' W). Your entire route around the valley can be studied from this outcropping.

Continue south until you reach SR 691, where there is a campsite along the road and space to park (2.4/2,528). Turn right and follow the road for about 2.5 miles, much of it an ascent along Devils Hole Mountain. The road meets the trailhead for yellow-blazed Long Mountain Trail on the right (4.9/2,934). This path covers the 8.7 miles along the western side of the route.

Initially, Long Mountain Trail follows a wide, level, grassy old road. It changes to a footpath and descends toward the drainage on the west side of Long Mountain itself before meeting the purple-blazed trail leading to Trout Pond (6.5/2,381). Past this intersection, Long Mountain Trail continues along an old road grade for several very easy miles. Note the area's odd topography. While there are several creeks running into the valley, their water is swallowed by the sinkholes you'll note as you pass. The trail climbs again, bears right, and eventually crests Cherry Ridge (11.8/2,061). A sharp, switchbacked descent from this ridge takes you down to Trout Run itself, which is bridged just a short distance from Trout Run Valley Road (13.6/1,455).

The orange blazes of Bucktail Trail appear immediately across the road. Follow them for a few hundred yards. The trail takes you through a large, circular parking lot, then to a trail kiosk behind a gate (complete with a sign and a bench) for Bucktail Trail on the right (13.8/1,538). Continue following the orange blazes. The trail seems to continue at a clearing but instead takes a sharp left. Keep your eye out for the pink-blazed Bucktail Cut Off Trail, which you'll follow as it veers off on the right.

For the next 3 miles, the trail traverses the south face of Halfmoon Mountain, dipping in and out of hollows as you go. This pleasant stretch of trail brings you to Halfmoon Run and the campsite there (16.5/1,925). Just above the campsite, turn onto yellow-blazed Halfmoon Trail, which begins a

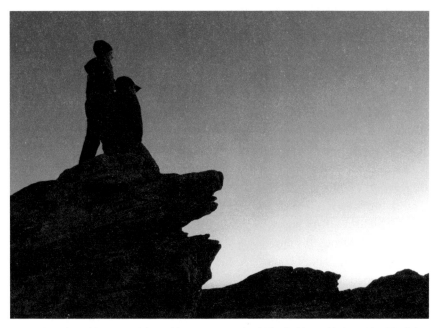

A couple enjoys the sunset from the craggy peak of Big Schloss, high on the Virginia-West Virginia border.

steady climb of about 600 feet up to a saddle between Great North Mountain (right) and Halfmoon Mountain (left) (17.5/2,547). This climb is steep and rocky at times, but the trail is well graded.

At the top of the saddle, the yellow-blazed trail continues to the right toward Tuscarora Trail. You'll pass that way soon, but first walk the 0.8 mile out and back (1.6 miles total) to reach Halfmoon Lookout, one of the most rewarding outlooks on the trip. To get there, take a left onto white-blazed Halfmoon Lookout Trail, which follows the lip of the saddle for about 0.5 mile where you reach the intersection, on the right, with pink-blazed German Wilson Trail (17.8/2,557). Bear left, continuing to follow the white blazes. Over the last few hundred yards, the trail ascends very steeply to the mountain's rocky summit (18.2/2,822). Note the stone foundations of an old fire lookout tower.

At the rocky crest of Halfmoon Lookout, take time to enjoy the panoramic view of the valley. On the right you'll see the ridge of Long Mountain, reaching south. Tibbet Knob dominates the far end of the valley. On your right, you'll see Great North Mountain looming above you, with the rocky bluff of Big Schloss away in the distance, toward Wolf Gap.

Retrace your steps, following the white blazes until you reach the intersection of Halfmoon Lookout Trail and Halfmoon Trail. From here, follow the yellow blazes as they take you about 0.7 mile of easy walking to blue-blazed Tuscarora Trail (19.7/2,800). Sometimes called "Big Blue," the Tuscarora Trail is one of the major arteries of the region, linking up with the AT in Shenandoah and then again near Marysville, Pennsylvania.

Join Tuscarora Trail at an L-shaped intersection, with the Tuscarora continuing north on the left, and south straight ahead. Follow it straight. Passing over a few bridges crossing marshy ground, the rocky footpath climbs a little more than 1 mile to the ridgeline of Great North Mountain. Here, Tuscarora Trail intersects with Mill Mountain Trail (20.8/3,126). This is your last turn of any significance. Take the orange-blazed Mill Mountain Trail south.

The remaining 6 miles of the trip all follow this long ridge to Wolf Gap. There are some ups and downs, but many of these miles are quite easy, and they offer numerous views of the area, both to the east and west. Pass Sandy Spring (23.3/2,793), a marked overlook on the right, and Big Schloss Cutoff Trail on the left (24.0/2,747). Continue southbound (straight) and you'll soon see Big Schloss looming ahead of you. The trail will edge around it to the right and meet a marked spur trail (24.9/2,761) that will take you up to the top of the Schloss, with its scramble to a view of the surrounding mountains (25.3/2,964/38° 56.4832' N, 78° 39.9490' W).

Head south on Mill Mountain Trail, which quickly becomes a steepish descent into the Wolf Gap Recreation Area on an old road grade. Once you reach the campground, you should have no difficulty spotting your vehicle (27.0/2,242).

OTHER OPTIONS

The Great North Mountain area abounds in trails to explore, and the presence of Tuscarora Trail means that you can hike to your heart's content. Consider using the trails to the east of Great North Mountain to walk an expanded loop that might visit Little Schloss or White Rock Cliff. Conversely, if you're looking to break this circuit into two similar halves (each of about 13 miles), stage a shuttle with one vehicle stationed at the parking lot where Long Mountain Trail meets Bucktail Trail and the other at Wolf Gap.

NEARBY

Woodstock, Virginia, is the closest town and offers a number of restaurants and businesses catering to travelers on the interstate. If you can't find what you're looking for in Woodstock, your next best bet is Front Royal.

ADDITIONAL INFORMATION

Contact the George Washington and Jefferson National Forests' Ranger District at 540-984-4101 or online at fs.usda.gov/gwj.

3

PENNSYLVANIA

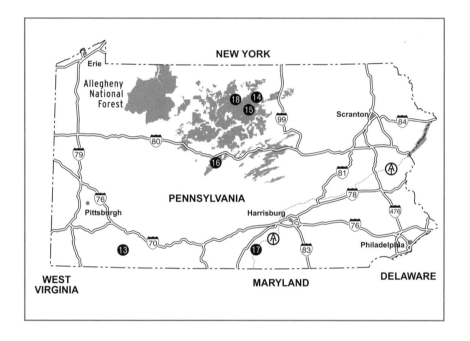

TRIP 13
BEAR WITH ME

Location: Bear Run Nature Reserve, Pennsylvania
Highlights: Beautiful rolling hills and creeks in the Laurel Highlands, vistas of the Youghiogheny River
Distance: 14.3 miles round-trip
Total Elevation Gain/Loss: 2,726 gain/2,726 loss
Trip Length: 2–3 days
Difficulty: Moderate
Recommended Maps and Other Resources:
- Western Pennsylvania Conservancy, *Bear Run Nature Preserve*, June 2010. www.paconserve.org/assets/2010_Bear_Run.pdf.
- USGS Quad: Mill Run.

Bear Run Nature Reserve offers a rich variety of landscapes, from dramatic views of the Youghiogheny River, to picturesque trails meandering through thickets of rhododendron, and beautiful valleys following Laurel Run and Bear Run. For the most part, its trails are gently graded and well marked, many of its stream crossings are bridged, and one is never too far away from the trailhead in case something goes awry. This makes Bear Run an excellent introduction to backpacking and the trails of Pennsylvania.

HIKE OVERVIEW

Easily walked in a weekend, the Bear Run Nature Reserve is an ideal destination for beginner backpackers wanting to practice for longer trips. After arriving at the trailhead, you'll enjoy a short and easy walk into the beautiful campsite where Hemlock Trail meets Bear Run. Saturday morning, you're off to explore most of the trails on the west side of the park, ending with the pleasant group sites along Snowbunny Trail. For Sunday, you'll have saved the best views for last. With an early start, you can walk around the Youghiogheny Peninsula and reach the vehicles in plenty of time to visit Fallingwater.

HOW TO REACH THE TRAILHEAD

From the Baltimore/Washington, D.C., area, head west on I-70, then follow I-68 into western Maryland. Take Exit 14B and head west on US 40. After about 20 miles, turn right on PA 381. You'll pass through Ohiopyle. Continue north. Just past the turnoff sign for Fallingwater, you'll see a sign for the trailhead on the right.

From Pittsburgh, take I-76 south until you reach Exit 75 for US 119/PA 66. Follow US 119 south to Connellsville. In Connellsville, turn left onto East Crawford Lane, then make a sharp left onto PA 711/Snyder Street. After about 8 miles, this road bends south and becomes PA 381/Mill Run Road. The trailhead parking lot is on your left in about 7 miles (39° 54.3644' N, 79° 27.5986' W). If you see the entrance to Fallingwater, stop and turn around, as you've gone too far.

The spacious trailhead parking lot is located behind a remodeled barn. Note, as you pull in, that Tree Trail (blazed yellow) branches off to the left from the driveway to the parking lot. Wagon Trail (blazed red) heads into the woods from behind the trailhead kiosk.

OVERNIGHT OPTIONS

Backcountry camping within the Bear Run Nature Reserve is limited to four designated campsites, which are available to backpackers on a first-come, first-served basis. When you pull into the parking lot, visit the trail kiosk, fill out a form, and place it in the cubby for the campsite(s) you want.

Given the restrictions on camping in the reserve (as well as how close the campsites are to one another), you'll have to plan your route carefully to make sure you arrive at one of the designated campsites in good time. The route in this book stops at the two best campsites over two days of fairly gentle walking.

Hemlock Trail Campsite (1.0/1,603/39° 53.915' N, 79° 27.253' W). This pretty little campsite is located alongside a creek and can be reached by walking into the park on Wagon and Ridge trails and turning right on Hemlock Trail. Unfortunately, there is space for just a few shelters. Arrive early to make sure you can secure space at this campsite.

Ridge Trail Campsite (leave route at 6.1/2,121/39° 54.549' N, 79° 26.006' W). The least attractive of the four campsites, this spot is little more than a small fire ring just off the trail with some flat space around it. If you choose to camp here, head south from the four-way intersection of Bear Run, Rhododendron, Tulip, and Ridge trails to follow Ridge Trail south about 0.4 mile to the campsite.

Lower Snowbunny Trail Campsite (7.3/1,793/39° 54.623' N, 79° 26.739' W). Just after you turn north at the intersection of Snowbunny and Rhododendron trails, you'll cross a bridge over a creek and soon see this large, well-marked

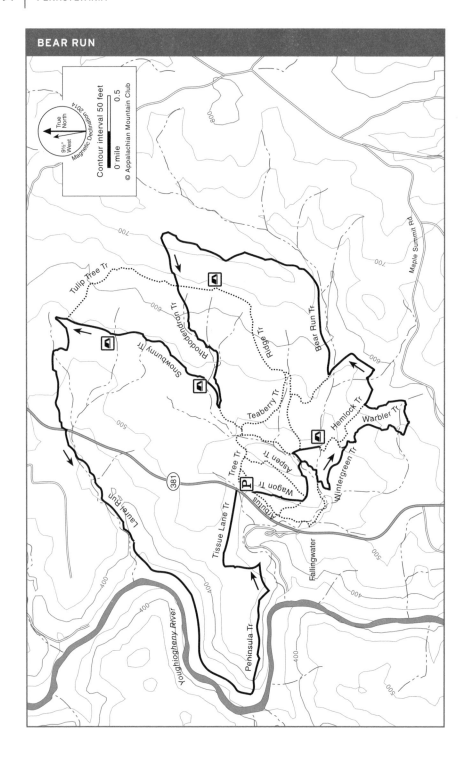

BEAR RUN

group site on your left. With easy access to water, several built-up fire rings, and enough space for quite a few tents, this campsite is the best in the reserve.

Upper Snowbunny Trail Campsite (8.1/1,818/39° 55.175' N, 79° 26.406' W). About 0.8 miles north along Snowbunny Trail after the first group site, you'll find another, very similar, campsite. Though it is smaller than the Lower Snowbunny site, it can certainly accommodate a number of shelters. It also has access to water.

HIKE DESCRIPTION

First, a few words of caution before you leave the trailhead. While the trails in Bear Run are well marked and generally well blazed, there are quite a lot of them, especially in the southeastern quadrant of the map. There are also quite a few unmarked trails intersecting with the established ones, and you'll also find that some of the well-established trails may be closed. Keep your map handy as you reach intersections, and be careful to keep your eye out for the blazes—remember that a double blaze means, "Pay attention!" and often signals that the trail is about to turn. Though it is quite possible to make a wrong turn, you should be able to reorient yourself and get back on track.

From the trailhead, you'll have a short walk of just 1 mile before reaching the campsite on Hemlock Trail. Take the red-blazed Wagon Trail southward from the far end of the parking lot. Soon this trail will intersect with Ridge Trail (0.3/1,565). Take a left and follow it past an intersection with Arbutus Trail on the right (a little stone staircase). You'll reach an intersection with Hemlock Trail (0.84/1,634). Take a right on Hemlock Trail and walk the remaining few hundred yards to the Hemlock Trail Campsite, overlooking Bear Run (1.0/1,603).

On day two, retrace your steps to Ridge Trail and take a left. Ridge Trail descends westward until it intersects with Arbutus Trail (1.25/1,584). There, take another left. At this point you'll be following the outer periphery of the reserve. First, you'll pass through a region of the forest carpeted by rhododendron and cross a bridge over a babbling creek. Turn left on Wintergreen Trail (1.45/1,517) and then right on Warbler Trail (2.0/1,683). Warbler Trail takes a number of left-hand turns that you could miss because there are other forest tracks; keep your eyes on the blazes. Take a right-hand turn on Hemlock Trail (3.1/1,906).

The path starts to get a bit more difficult on Hemlock Trail. At one point, the trail dips down steeply to a tributary of Bear Run and climbs sharply above it. Keep your eyes open for the blazes, as there are a number of unmarked footpaths at the top of the gully. If you find yourself at a loss, look to the left as you climb out of the streambed as the trail takes a hard turn (3.35/1,994). Eventually, Hemlock Trail will join up with Bear Run Trail at a V-shaped intersection that you can recognize by the fire ring (3.77/1,821). (Note that this is not a designated campsite, however.)

Turn right on Bear Run Trail and begin the only notable ascent of the trip as you walk 1.9 miles and climb 700 feet to the top of a ridge, the highest point on the circuit (2,478). The path follows an old road, so the grade is gentle enough. You should have lots of opportunities to enjoy views of the creek below you and to the right. Eventually, the trail tops out on a broad ridgeline. If the leaves are off the trees, you'll have partial views of the surrounding Laurel Highlands.

After following this ridgeline for a few tenths of a mile, the trail turns west and gets serious about losing altitude. The walk down is never especially steep or tricky, however, and will probably feel rather pleasant after the climb up Bear Run Trail. You'll soon reach a four-way trail junction, where Bear Run, Ridge, Tulip Tree, and Rhododendron trails come together (6.1/2,121). Continue straight on Rhododendron Trail, and about 1 mile later, take a sharp right on to Snowbunny Trail (7.06/1,711). Lower Snowbunny Trail Campsite is on the left, just after the little bridge (7.3/1,793). If this site is full, you'll need to continue about 0.8 mile farther up Snowbunny Trail to the Upper Snowbunny Trail Campsites, marked by a bridge over a small creek (8.1/1,818).

After striking camp on day three, you have about 7 miles to walk and some of the best scenery of the trip to enjoy. Head north along Snowbunny Trail, and arrive at the three-way junction with Laurel Run Trail (8.6/1,795). Turn left. Over the next 2.1 miles, the trail descends gradually about 600 feet, following Laurel Run as it flows past PA 381 and toward the Youghiogheny. Unlike much of the trail so far, the footing here becomes rocky and fractured in spots, so watch your step. At one point, the trail climbs up slightly to an open area and acts as if it might emerge from the woods and into a farmer's fields (9.3/1,618). Instead, bear left and continue following Laurel Run Trail until it reaches PA 381 (9.5/1,477).

After the road crossing, Laurel Run Trail draws nearer to the run again. This area can become a bit boggy before the trail crosses the run and begins following it on the left. Although the trail never really climbs much, the run starts to fall away beneath you to the right and the ridge becomes more pronounced on your left. Soon enough, you will cross a sidehill with views of the Youghiogheny River Gorge on your right.

If you're paying attention to your map, you'll expect Laurel Run Trail to turn into Peninsula Trail. Instead, the trails on this side of PA 381 are all effectively one. You won't notice any transition. When you make the sharp,

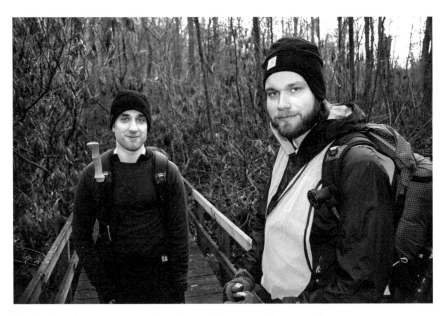

Two backpackers pause for a break on a bridge spanning Bear Run.

eastward turn at the far end of the peninsula, the ground gets a bit rougher than what you've enjoyed so far in Bear Run. There's a steep descent or two and one steep climb as you approach two overlooks.

As you walk along this section of the trail, keep your eye out for the first overlook, which is not marked on the official Western Pennsylvania Conservancy map. You'll be heading down a steeper grade and need to turn hard right to reach an open cliff overlooking the river gorge (12.2/1,295). Take your time and enjoy this spot, as it is the most open vista on the trail. Paradise Overlook, a little farther along the trail, overlooks a bend in the Youghiogheny, but is a little too grown in to be spectacular (12.8/1,299).

From Paradise Overlook, walk on for a few tenths of a mile to reach one of the parking lots for Fallingwater. The trail turns left immediately before this lot (13.1/1,367), climbs moderately, makes a sharp right (13.7/1,513), and follows a dirt road eastward to the trailhead parking lot on the opposite side of PA 381. You won't see a sign for Tissue Lane Trail marked on the map (or at least I didn't). Just keep walking eastward down the dirt road and you'll reach your vehicle (14.3/1,506).

OTHER OPTIONS

While the terrain at Bear Run is too gentle to serve as the backdrop for a strenuous weekend of backpacking, an intermediate backpacker could circumnavigate the park by walking the following trails: Arbutus, Wintergreen, Warbler, Hemlock, Bear Run, Rhododendron, Snowbunny, Laurel Run, Peninsula, Tissue, Tree, and Rhododendron, and camp at the group site on Snowbunny. The next day, climb Rhododendron Trail to the intersection with Ridge Trail and descend to the vehicles or, more aggressively, follow Bear Run Trail and work your way back around.

If you're feeling more conservative about the mileage, you might consider base camping for two nights at one of the three better campsites and day-hiking the eastern and western halves of the reserve.

NEARBY

One of the best reasons to take a weekend and backpack Bear Run is the proximity of Frank Lloyd Wright's celebrated Fallingwater, a National Historical Landmark that is often listed as one of the greatest works of American architecture. As you hike along the southern extremity of Peninsula Trail, you'll pass the parking lot for the house. To visit, you'll need to purchase a ticket. More information can be had at Fallingwater's site: fallingwater.org. If you find that you have the time, another Wright house, Kentuck Knob, is situated south of Ohiopyle. See Kentuck Knob's website at kentuckknob.com.

Ohiopyle itself attracts quite a crowd of whitewater rafters and kayakers. You can expect to find a variety of pubs, restaurants, hotels, and stores catering to outdoorspeople. You'll have no trouble finding a pleasant place to enjoy a post-hike meal or a store to help you replace a forgotten piece of equipment.

ADDITIONAL INFORMATION

The Western Pennsylvania Conservancy owns Bear Run Nature Reserve. Guidelines for visiting the reserve may be found at www.paconserve. org/assets/2010_WPC_Property_Visitor_Guidelines.pdf. For additional information about the reserve, please call 724-329-7803.

TRIP 14
RIM TO RIM TO RIM

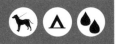

Location: Tioga State Forest, Pennsylvania
Highlights: Vistas of Pine Creek Gorge and the Allegheny Plateau
Distance: 30 miles one-way
Total Elevation Gain/Loss: 5,499 feet of gain/5,167 feet of loss
Trip Length: 2–4 days
Difficulty: Challenging
Recommended Maps and Other Resources:
- Chuck Dillon, *Guide to the West Rim Trail*, 4th ed. Wellsboro, PA: Pine Creek Press, 2012.
- Pennsylvania's Department of Conservation and Natural Resource, *West Rim Trail Map*, dcnr.state.pa.us/forestry/recreation/hiking/ stateforesttrails/westrimtrail/.
- USGS Quads: Tiadaghton and Cedar Run.

Pennsylvania's Pine Creek Gorge contrasts sharply with the surrounding peaceful farmland, plunging 800 feet to the river below and spanning 2,000 feet from rim to rim, to the shock and enjoyment of its many visitors. West Rim Trail (WRT) offers backpackers an excellent opportunity to explore this striking natural feature, following the lip of the gorge for mile after mile of fine vistas and beautiful forests.

HIKE OVERVIEW

Covering 30 miles along the west rim of Pine Creek Gorge, WRT is a point-to-point route that begins at the trail's south terminus near Rattlesnake Rock and heads north to Ansonia, Pennsylvania. Along the way, the trail passes a total of eighteen vistas, numerous opportunities for fine backcountry camping, and a wide variety of forest environments. Although its forests were clear-cut in the late nineteenth and early twentieth centuries, the existing, maturing forests are diverse and stunning.

WRT will interest backpackers with varying levels of experience. While the route does feature some ups and downs, it is well blazed, excellently maintained, and fairly gentle. It offers an opportunity to expand trip range and build endurance, while enjoying a beautiful and rewarding trail.

HOW TO REACH THE TRAILHEAD

From Williamsport, Pennsylvania, head west on US 220. Keep right to head north on US 15, toward Mansfield. After about 27 miles, take the exit for PA 414, and take a left. Bear right onto PA 287 in the town of Morris, then head about 11 miles to Wellsboro. Turn left onto Main Street, which becomes PA 660 and PA 362 as it continues west. About 8 miles outside of Wellsboro, take a left on US 6. You have two options for reaching the trailhead and establishing a shuttle.

If you prefer to establish your own shuttle, take a left on Forest Road in Ansonia; this brings you to the northern terminus of WRT just a few hundred yards past the intersection with US 6 (41° 44.354' N, 77° 25.984' W). After dropping off a vehicle, return to Wellsboro and then head south on PA 287 to Morris. Bear right on PA 414, which will take you to the canyon in about 8 miles. On the left you'll see a signed parking lot for the southern terminus of WRT (41° 32.4333' N, 77° 24.3472' W).

Pine Creek Outfitters (570-724-3003) also offers a shuttle service to the southern terminus of WRT. To reach the outfitter, continue 1 mile farther on US 6 through Ansonia and you'll spot their establishment on the left. You'll merely need to walk the extra 1 mile from the northern terminus to your vehicle when you finish the route.

OVERNIGHT OPTIONS

Camping is permitted along WRT. Permits are not required unless staying in one place for more than one night; for purposes of safety, however, you may request a free permit from Tioga State Forest. Contact them for the latest information regarding campfires; fires are usually permitted, but they are banned during periods of high wildfire hazard. Limit your group size to ten. You'll have no difficulty locating excellent campsites along WRT, though in a few places water availability is an issue.

Lloyds Run (0.4/963/41° 32.663' N, 77° 24.311' W). If you're coming in late, look for these campsites on the right before you start the long climb up Lloyds Run. Many tent sites have easy access to water.

Bohen Run (4.15/1,485/41° 34.635' N, 77° 24.110' W). A few nice tent sites are here, but Bohen Run is especially noteworthy for being the last reliable water source for the next 9 miles of the trail. If you're hiking in dry conditions, be sure to fill up here.

Gundigut Hollow (8.4/2,009/41° 36.588' N, 77° 25.391' W). If your bottles are full, then it makes excellent sense to camp at this broad site high above Pine Creek.

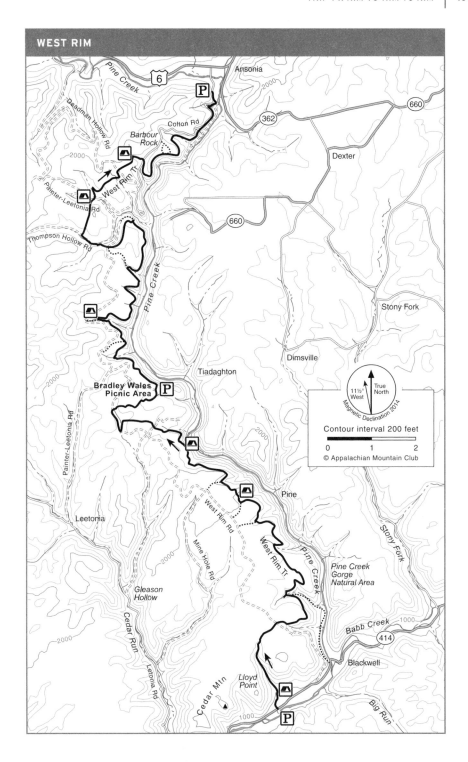

Good Springs Hollow (10.7/1,644/41° 37.562' N, 77° 26.856' W). Just before the vista marking the descent into this hollow, there is a campsite with a fire ring under a stand of evergreens. Bring your water or descend to the run to fill up.

Little Slate Run (17.4/1,562/41° 39.962' N, 77° 29.018' W). The trail rides high above this hollow, then descends to meet the run at one of the most beautiful spots along the trail. This is an ideal spot to spend the night or just take an afternoon break.

Painter-Leetonia Road (24.2/1,627/41° 42.351' N, 77° 29.125' W). About 6 miles from the end of the trail, this popular site sees a lot of traffic and is near the road. You might prefer a more backcountry camping spot.

Bear Run (25.9/1,784/41° 43.094' N, 77° 28.074' W). An idyllic little site sitting in an open meadow along this run, Bear Run is also one of the last likely campsites along WRT. If you cross the run, you'll find more tenting sites downstream.

HIKE DESCRIPTION

Cross PA 414, look for the orange blazes, and begin walking along the shady eastern bank of Lloyds Run. Sign in at the trail register and pass the campsites on your right. In short order, the trail climbs the run toward the Allegheny Plateau (0.5/1,000), following an old grade. The trail is not especially steep, but it is a steady climb of about 800 feet over 1.3 miles. Toward the top, it leaves the run, steepens, and turns right, passing over flat ground at the top of the plateau. Cross West Rim Road (2.4/1,857) and come upon your first vista, looking southward into Pine Creek Gorge (3.13/1,802).

As you turn and begin walking north, WRT begins the soon-to-be familiar pattern of dropping down gently to meet a run, then climbing and often rounding an eastward-looking promontory to regain the plateau. Level walking ensues until you reach the next gully. In this manner, the trail takes you north along the canyon's west rim. At Bohen Run (4.15/1,485), top off your bottles, especially if the weather has been dry. Some of the other runs may have water in them, but the next certain source of water could be as far as 9 miles ahead.

WRT continues northward along the plateau, where mountain laurel sometimes grows in thick around the trail, then reaches Dillon Hollow (6.07/1,678) and Steel Hollow (7.35/1,722). In Steel Hollow, note a yellow-blazed trail that allows quick access to West Rim Road if you should need to leave WRT. Similar access trails may be found in the next two hollows: Pine Trail (8.2/1,945) and Gundigut Trail (8.86/1,886).

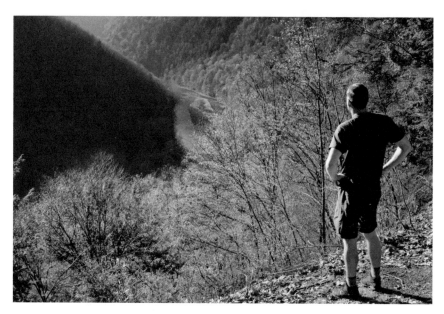

A backpacker greets the dawn over Pennsylvania's grand canyon from West Rim Trail.

WRT leaves these access trails behind, climbs from the hollow, and begins exploring a more isolated stretch of the canyon's rim. After reaching the campsite and vista just south of Good Spring Hollow (10.7/1,644), the trail drops down into the run and climbs steadily away from the canyon. The path wanders through a forest of beech, aspen, and hemlock before meeting West Rim Road (12.7/1,722). Turn right on the road, and follow it for about 0.6 mile. The trail takes a sharp bend to the right, reenters the forest, and crosses a boggy area where there is a reliable spring (13.3/1,784).

After descending slightly, WRT edges along a few clearings, then bends left to reach the Bradley Wales Picnic Area. At the midpoint of the trail, this area offers water, toilets, and vehicle access (14.6/1,620). Beyond this point, the trail approaches the canyon rim for a series of vistas of the gorge (14.7/1,627). North of these overlooks, the path dives to meet Ice Break Run (16/1,504) and Little Slate Run (17.3/1,581), each of which has an access trail leading to Painter-Leetonia Road. From there, the gullies come fast as the trail dips down into Tumbling Run, Horse Run, and Burdick Run (19.8/1,572). (Burdic Run offers a shortcut: its yellow-blazed Siemens Trail cuts off about 2 miles of walking along WRT as it extends northward toward Colton Point, then returns southward.)

From Burdic Run, WRT climbs again to regain the plateau, then enjoys some easy walking along an old grade through a forest of beech and birch. As the trail bends west, the path suddenly turns left to climb uphill, while yellow-blazed Refuge Trail continues straight along the road grade (21.4/1,634); this turn is easily missed. From the junction, WRT climbs about 250 vertical feet southward, then descends fairly sharply before reaching Thompson Hollow Road (22.6/1,542). Here, the left branch of Four Mile Run offers plenty of water and a pleasant place for a break. Walk westward along this road, but keep an eye out for the trail's right-hand turn (23.2/1,643). The path climbs stiffly about 300 feet and redescends before crossing the road again. A little bridge spans the right branch of Four Mile Run (24.2/1,614).

The trail passes campsites along the creek to the left as it ascends gently along a logging road. After passing a gate, the trail turns sharply right (24.4/1,705) and follows a more open ridge. It crosses Deadman Hollow Road (named for a trapper who froze to death in the early twentieth century; 25.3/1,877) and descends gently to Bear Run and the camping there (25.9/1,783).

The trail soon crosses Colton Road (26.2/1,733), enters a pine plantation, and follows the canyon rim very closely for about 1.5 miles. The rim bends eastward over this stretch and offers numerous grand views of Pine Creek Gorge. Mind your footing; the trail is often quite close to impressively sheer dropoffs.

For the next 2 miles, WRT descends steadily toward the northern terminus, its route coinciding more and more with an old logging grade. You've nearly reached the trail's end when it crosses Owassie Road (29.6/1,332). Soon after, you'll arrive at the trail register and the trailhead parking lot across from a forestry maintenance building (30/1,198).

If your vehicle is parked at Pine Creek Outfitters, continue walking north from the northern terminus along Forest Road and take a left on US 6. You'll reach the turnoff for the outfitter in about 1 mile, on the left.

OTHER OPTIONS

Several link trails connect WRT with other trails in this region of Pennsylvania. About 1.9 miles from the southern terminus of the trail, Long Branch Trail connects to Black Forest Trail. Around 4.1 miles from the southern terminus, another connector runs down Bohen Run to join up with Mid State Trail.

If you're looking to walk a shorter trip, many backpackers choose to be shuttled south to the Bradley Wales Picnic Area and then walk north to the northern terminus. This option allows you to cut about half the miles from the trail while still visiting most of its best vistas.

NEARBY

Wellsboro is the largest town in the area and offers a number of restaurants and diners. If you can't find what you're looking for in Wellsboro, either look along PA 414, where many businesses cater to outdoorspeople, or return to Williamsport.

ADDITIONAL INFORMATION

For more information, contact Pennsylvania Tioga State Forest, online at dcnr.state.pa.us/forestry/stateforests/tioga or by phone at 570-724-2868.

TRIP 15
WHICH WAY TO MUNICH?

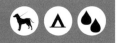

Location: Tiadaghton State Forest, Pennsylvania

Highlights: Vistas of Pine Creek Gorge and the Allegheny Plateau, rich northern hardwood forests, and one of the most demanding trails in the region

Distance: 42 miles round-trip

Total Elevation Gain/Loss: 8,807 feet gain/8,807 feet loss

Trip Length: 2–6 days

Difficulty: Strenuous

Recommended Maps and Other Resources:

- Chuck Dillon, *The Black Forest Trail: A Backpacker's Interpretive Guide*. Wellsboro, PA: Pine Creek Press, 2008. The map that ships with this book is the best available.
- USGS Quads: Slate Run, Lee Fire Tower, Cedar Run, and Cammal.

The Black Forest Trail (BFT)—with its sharp elevation gain, convoluted route, and wild succession of ups and downs—demands a great deal from those seeking to walk it, but it gives a great deal too. No other single trail captures so much of the essence of Pennsylvania's great hiking—the varied terrain; the vistas of gorges carved deep into the plateau; the close, steep hollows; the quaint villages. This is the one Pennsylvania loop that every backpacker in the region must hike, but come prepared: it's no mere walk in the woods.

HIKE OVERVIEW

While the BFT is most commonly hiked counterclockwise from Slate Run, Pennsylvania, this route describes it as a clockwise loop that heads south from town. Either way is defensible, but the clockwise route tackles the toughest hiking (in the loop's southeast quadrant) first, sets you up for easier miles later in the trip (on the trail's west and north sides), and concludes with the exhilarating descent into Slate Run. Whichever way you walk it, however, the BFT will test your resolve and your resilience. Some have called it the toughest trail in Pennsylvania, or even the Mid-Atlantic. Such judgments are subjective, but the BFT is a worthy backpacking challenge.

HOW TO REACH THE TRAILHEAD

For most of the East Coast, Williamsport will be the gateway to the superb backpacking in north-central Pennsylvania. From Williamsport, head west on US 220 for about 15 miles, then take Exit 120 for PA 44 north. Turn right and proceed north about 12.5 miles. Bear right to continue onto PA 414. About 14 miles later, you'll reach the little town of Slate Run. Turn left sharply and cross Pine Creek over the bridge. Continue northeast on Slate Run Road. You'll spot a parking bay on the right amid a plantation of pines (41° 28.518' N, 77° 30.722' W). A short trail leads downhill to the BFT. If this bay is full, there is a parking lot about 2 miles up the road, also with easy access to the trail (albeit 2 miles farther along the trail, clockwise).

OVERNIGHT OPTIONS

With abundant backcountry sites to choose from, the BFT is a backpacker's dream. You'll be hard pressed to find a section of trail without an attractive campsite, often near water. A few even boast excellent views nearby. Tiadaghton State Forest strongly recommends that, for safety reasons, you request a permit for tent camping, though they are not required. The permits are free of charge.

Slate Run (0.0/767/41° 28.413' N, 77° 30.486' W). If you're arriving late and are looking for a quick place to pitch and catch some sleep, there are a few campsites on the southern side of the Slate Run crossing. From the trail register near the parking bay, take a right and walk a few hundred yards to the river.

Naval Run (11.7/946/41° 27.796' N, 77° 31.437' W). After the 1,200-foot descent to reach Naval Run, you may want to camp before taking on the steep climb out of this narrow valley. If so, you're in luck: there are several campsites available. Look for the flat shelf on your right as you walk up the road grade on the southern side of the creek. There's also a lovely site with a view at the very top of the climb from the run (13/2,088), though it's dry.

Callahan Run (15.5/989/41° 26.925' N, 77° 32.068' W). As you bottom out the descent along Callahan Run, the trail crosses a tributary before climbing again. You'll spot a few attractive, but rather narrow, campsites alongside the creek.

Baldwin Branch (19.6/1,731/41° 27.585' N, 77° 35.191' W). On the western side of the BFT, where there's a hollow, there's usually a good campsite with water. Expect to find tent sites where the BFT dips down to join Baldwin Branch, where the trail climbs out of this long hollow (21/1,912), and again at the next hollow 3 miles farther along the plateau, tucked in a rhododendron thicket (24.1/1,808).

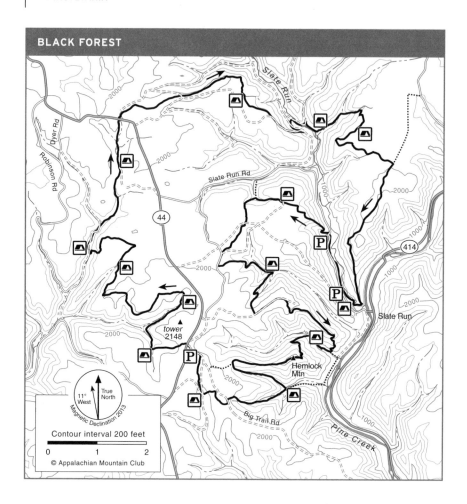

County Line Run (26.2/1,437/41° 29.228' N, 77° 36.677' W). There are plenty of campsites nearby after the tricky rock scrambling needed to descend to County Line Run. Some sites are just on the far side of the run; you'll come upon others as you walk up the run. There is also an ideal spot just north of the hunters' camp (28.1/1,874) toward the top of the branch. Water is plentiful.

Red Run (35/1,106/41° 31.367' N, 77° 31.200' W). As you leave Slate Run and prepare for one last climb, you'll find several appealing campsites along the run's lower reaches. If you happen to be there in summer, these sites are within a short walk from several swimming holes along Slate Run. A few sites are also perched on the plateau above the run, but you'll need to carry water up the climb.

HIKE DESCRIPTION

The BFT is beautiful, but demanding, and does not give up its charms easily. As one backpacking friend of mine put it, the trail "wanders around a plateau, looking for gullies to dive into." You'll get a sense for the truth of that statement as you walk the 19 miles of the trail's southeast quadrant, the trail's most difficult section.

From the trailhead, turn left after the registry, and start following the orange blazes. For the next 1.75 miles, you'll be walking along the left bank of Slate Run, alternating between a road grade and a narrower footpath. The trail climbs up to the road, crosses it (1.83/983), and starts working its way along a rocky ridgeline (2.29/1,450). The valley of Slate Run opens out behind you before the trail reaches the plateau, passes by a hunters' cabin (3.24/1,848), and then descends into Fosters Run. In wet weather, the trail and the creek may be colocated, but the blazes will lead you onward.

From the bottom of Fosters Run (3.89/1,465), turn left and climb to regain the plateau, cross a forest track (4.5/1,858), and then walk briefly along another road before the trail reenters the forest on the left (5.6/1,949). The BFT now dives into the picturesque valley of Little Slate Run; a sidehill descent will take you past a few campsites on the right side of the run (6.86/1,281). Over the next 2 miles, the BFT climbs about 800 feet onto a ridgeline pointing toward Pine Creek.

When it crests this ridge (8.3/2,101), the trail intersects the blue-blazed Baldwin Gas Line Trail, which leads westward to PA 44 (if you want to walk a shorter loop, this trail would enable you to cut off the southern half of this route). The BFT heads easterly (left) and is at first flat. A number of short spur trails lead to a few named viewpoints. Soon, though, it starts a precipitous descent into Naval Run. Keep your eyes out for blazes, as there are a few occasions where you could get off-trail. After you cross Naval Run (11.2/841), head upstream (right) on an old grade. About 1 mile later, the BFT starts one of its most sustained climbs, gaining about 1,000 feet over 1.3 miles. When you reach the top of Hemlock Mountain (13/2,096), you'll be treated to more fine vistas, then you'll walk west along the mountain's backbone.

The BFT is far from finished with its diving and climbing. Just shy of PA 44, the trail turns left to dive into Callahan Run's gully (14.2/1,871). Be careful: this rugged descent is confusingly blazed at times. You'll know that you're almost to the bottom when the trail sidehills a few dozen yards above the run. Cross the creek (15.5/989), and climb about 1,100 feet out of the valley, eventually reaching a road (17/2,097).

Fortunately, once you climb out of Callahan Run, easier walking follows on the western side of the plateau. Turn left and walk on the road for a spell, regain the woods on the right, pass a hunters' cabin, and cross another road (17.7/1,957). Then, after passing through a wood, take a left on Trout Run Road and arrive at PA 44 (18.9/2,069). From there, the trail will drop down into Baldwin Branch, where there is a campsite with easy access to water (19.6/1,731). The path sidehills within this gully for just under 2 miles, eventually being joined by a blue-blazed connector trail on the right before passing an old stone structure (20.9/1,843). The BFT then climbs back to the plateau (21.3/2,033). Three miles of easy walking, with occasional views westward, follow before you reach a narrow hollow shrouded in rhododendron (24/826).

Leave this hollow by the BFT's switchbacked old grade to the plateau, then pass through a clearing before regaining the forest. More easy miles will follow before the trail starts a rocky and precipitous descent into County Line Branch (26.1/1,423). After a few scrambling-style moves, follow switchbacks down to the creek. Cross it, and then follow the trail right. Over the next 3 miles, the path crosses the branch many, many times. Keep careful track of the blazes, as the trail flirts at times with an old grade: when in doubt, cross the creek. You'll soon come to a hunters' lodge (28/1,843). Pass in front of the cabin—note the blaze on the gateway—and then be treated to a rare BFT luxury: a little bridge. You'll pass shady campsites under the pines before reaching PA 44 once again (29/1,987). Glance left to see the sign for Potter County: "God's Country."

Cross PA 44, and turn right as the orange blazes take you down a few stairs and into the forest. Pay attention as you walk east as the trail does cross paths with blue-blazed Sentiero di Shay. The next 3.8 miles are easy, level walking, often with a game fence on your right. You'll cross a road, pass a small campsite with an unreliable stream, and begin a direct descent on a road grade (32.8/1,813), which ends at Francis Road (33.5/1,270). Here, the BFT bends back along the road for a few hundred yards, bears to the right into the forest, and drops down to a bridge over the river—a good spot for a break (34.6/1,073), though there are better ones a little farther along.

Follow the dirt road on the north side of Slate Run to pick up the path again. Soon the road becomes a footpath and crosses a beautiful creek and waterfall over a little bridge. Then, the BFT follows Red Run (34.9/1,068), passes a few campsites, and gives you a few more chances to get your feet wet. When the trail turns rightward (35.3/1,212), you'll know that you're beginning the last, steepest, and most technical climb on the BFT. Over the next 0.9

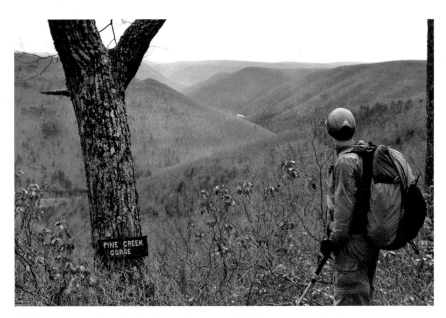

A hiker surveys Pine Creek Gorge from one of BFT's many overlooks.

mile, you'll gain about 700 feet, much of it over rocky terrain where the blazes merely suggest where you might think of going next. Still, the climb is rewarding: the waterworks on your left are fetching, and the trail tops out on the plateau with a rocky prominence where you can survey your route and catch your breath (36.2/1,867).

Other views follow as the orange blazes take you southbound over this plateau. The walking is exceptionally easy here, but it is possible to lose the trail in the thick foliage. When you arrive at the turnoff for Algerine Trail (which takes you to West Rim Trail) on the left (38.1/1,986), bear hard right and pass a rather suspect water source before the BFT descends on the plateau's right flank (39.3/2,060). Right away, you'll enjoy vistas of Pine Creek Gorge (40/1,678), then you'll pass the remains of the old slate quarry. If you have a sharp eye, you can spot the pine plantation below where your vehicle is parked.

While an old road grade continues straight (offering a high-water route if Slate Run is dangerous), the trail turns right (40.7/1,224) and descends sharply down a ridgeline dominated by slate formations before it veers right and side-hills down to Slate Run (41.4/754). Do be careful crossing the creek, as it is potentially dangerous, though usually it will just get you wet below the knees. On the far side, pass through the campsites and follow the old railroad grade back to the trail register and the end of your journey (42/859).

OTHER OPTIONS

If you're not quite ready to thru-hike the BFT, the intersections with PA 44 at the center of the loop make it comparatively easy to stage shuttles and hike the trail by halves. Additionally, the trail's rather peculiar shape means that there are a number of cutoff trails, which allow you to customize which sections of the trail you want to walk and which you don't. The yellow-blazed trail cutting off the "extra" descent and climb out of Callahan Run likely sees heavy traffic.

Note that if you get into trouble in the BFT's southeastern quadrant, there are trails at the bottom of many of the runs. They all lead to Pine Creek and civilization.

For those hungry for more hiking, the BFT is only one course among many in this part of Pennsylvania. The North and South Link trails connect westward with the Susquehannock Trail System, and Algerine Trail connects northward to West Rim Trail. It's possible for the ambitious backpacker to walk hundreds of miles on the Allegheny Plateau.

NEARBY

Williamsport is the nearest large town, but the roads along Pine Creek (PA 44 and PA 414) are lined with businesses serving the sports- and outdoorspeople who frequent this area. You'll have no difficulty finding a hotel, bar, restaurant, gas station, or general store willing to serve grubby backpackers.

ADDITIONAL INFORMATION

For more information about the BFT, you may visit the Tiadaghton State Forest at its website, dcnr.state.pa.us/forestry/stateforests/tiadaghton, or call 570-753-5409.

TRIP 16
FRONT AND CENTER:
THE ALLEGHENY FRONT TRAIL

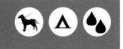

Location: Moshannon State Forest, Pennsylvania
Highlights: Views from the Allegheny Front, Six Mile Run, and Moshannon Creek
Distance: 39.6 miles round-trip
Total Elevation Gain/Loss: 5,470 feet gain/5,470 feet loss
Trip Length: 3–5 days
Difficulty: Moderate
Recommended Maps and Other Resources:
- *Allegheny Front Trail: Moshannon State Forest.* Department of Conservation and Natural Resources, Bureau of Forestry, 2010. (Contact the Pennsylvania Department of Conservation and Natural Resources for a free version of this map. Do be aware that even this map is inaccurate in spots, especially in the southwestern quadrant of the loop.)
- USGS Quads: Port Matilda, Black Moshannon, and Bear Knob.

Over its 40-mile course, the lovely Allegheny Front Trail (AFT) passes through remarkably varied terrain that includes mature hardwood forests, pine plantations, beautiful water courses like Six Mile Run and Black Moshannon Creek, the high exposed ridge of the front itself, and the swamps of Moss-Hanne Trail in Black Moshannon State Park. A walk along the AFT is also a walk through the history of human exploitation of these forests and subsequent efforts to reclaim the land. Moshannon Creek (sometimes called "Red Mo") runs red with the iron residue left over from coal mining, and the attentive hiker will find the crumbling ruins of camps and forges along the route.

HIKE OVERVIEW
A relatively new trail, the AFT was established in the 1990s when Ralph Seeley and members of the Keystone Trails Association, the Ridge and Valley Outings Club, the Penn State Outing Club, and the Quehanna Area Trails Club took up the cause. Five years later, the trail was completed. Seeley's name

is immortalized by the signs marking vistas along the Allegheny Front as "Ralph's Pretty Good View" and "Ralph's Majestic Vista."

The AFT is gaining in popularity rapidly, perhaps because it offers an excellent multiday backpacking trip that covers relatively easy ground without sacrificing rewarding vistas and a rich variety of environments. It is an excellent trip for an intermediate backpacker looking to walk a "big loop" and develop the skills and confidence needed for undertaking other adventures. Advanced backpackers will also find the AFT an enjoyable and pleasant circuit, especially in autumn when the foliage is at its height.

While the AFT is usually well blazed and signed, it does have its eccentricities. First, though it is often yellow blazed, it is sometimes orange blazed, and in a few sections, even red blazed. (If you take a look at the paint along Six Mile Run, you can see that the yellow paint covers originally orange blazes.) There are also a few places where the signage could be clearer, and you should be alert to sudden zigs and zags. The detailed description should help you avoid ending up somewhere you did not intend to be.

HOW TO REACH THE TRAILHEAD

Since the AFT is located squarely in the middle of Pennsylvania, the trailhead is easily reached from most of the eastern seaboard. From the Pennsylvania Turnpike, take I-99 north past Altoona. Take Exit 62 and follow US 322 north. After about 10 miles, turn right on PA 504. In about 6 miles, PA 504 will descend to a bridge over Six Mile Run. There is a pull off and a parking lot for several vehicles just on the near (west) side of the bridge (40° 54.5463' N, 78° 6.2725' W).

OVERNIGHT OPTIONS

Camping is permitted all along the AFT, with the exception of the stretch that is within Black Moshannon State Park; effectively, that means that you cannot backcountry camp along the 3.2-mile portion of the trail between Julian Pike and Shirks Road.

Moshannon Creek In the trail's northwestern quadrant, there are campsites virtually every time the AFT crosses a tributary of Moshannon Creek. Attractive sites include Tork Run (4.78/1,351/40° 57.037' N, 78° 05.850' W), Dry Hollow, and Potter Run (6.06/1,367/440° 57.409' N, 78° 04.620' W). Don't drink water taken directly from Moshannon Creek.

Black Moshannon Creek (9.74/1,657/40° 57.399' N, 78° 02.406' W). At mile 9, the AFT intersects Shingle Mill Trail. About a quarter-mile farther along, a rhododendron thicket hides two smallish campsites on the right. The

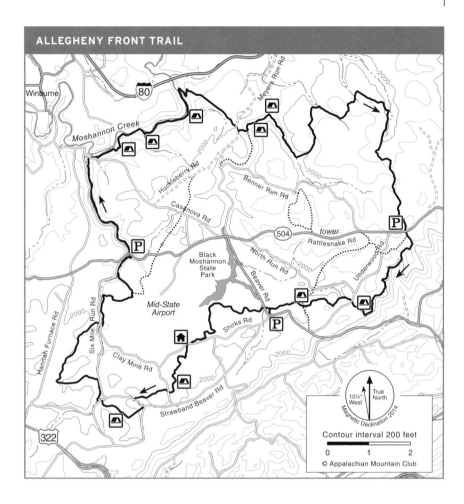

trail then reaches a hunting lodge where Benner Run and Black Moshannon Creek join. There is a third, broader campsite there.

Rock Run (16.2/2,078/40° 56.613' N, 77° 59.439' W). As the AFT follows Rock Run on its western side, you'll find a number of campsites near water.

Allegheny Front and Smays Run Just past PA 504, the AFT follows the ridgeline of the Allegheny Front with a series of impressive views. Where there is a view, there is usually a rough and ready campsite nearby. These sites are small, high, dry, and potentially chilly (21.3/2,117/40° 53.402' N, 77° 59.533' W). If you walk on to Smays Run, there is a broad site with water, but it is close to a road (23.8/1,899/40° 53.557' N, 78° 01.637' W).

Upper Shirks Road (30/1,903/40° 51.935' N, 78° 04.973' W). The AFT turns left at the lodge on Shirks Road (28.7/1,876) and follows a stream for 1.6 miles.

This area is sometimes marshy, with boardwalks in places, but there are a few campsites.

Upper Six Mile Run (32.2/1,887/40° 51.289' N, 78° 06.392' W). After mile 32, the AFT follows the high reaches of Six Mile Run for a spell. You'll spot a few very attractive campsites.

HIKE DESCRIPTION

From the parking lot, cross the bridge, and climb over the guardrail on the eastern bank of Six Mile Run. You should be able to spot the yellow-blazed trail closely following the bank of the run as it heads north. The first three miles of the trip are easy walking along this charming creek. Periodically, the trail will take a hard right and do some climbing alongside the run, but these little ascents and descents are fairly gentle.

You'll know that you've almost arrived at Casanova Road when the trail turns away from the creek and climbs a few hundred feet. The path will then lose much of the elevation it gained as it reaches the road. Turn right and walk along the road for just a few yards (2.9/1,428). The AFT diverges from the road to the left. Soon, it will turn uphill in a hollow (3.5/1,408), climb steadily, cut back to the left, and reach a prominence where there is a primitive (and dry) campsite (3.75/1,680). Just beneath this crest, a leftward path leads to an impressive view of Moshannon Creek.

Over the next several miles, you'll see signs of humankind's less than happy interaction with nature. Moshannon Creek owes its distinctive, striking red color to the iron compounds that pollute its water from the numerous old coal mines in its watershed. The AFT follows this river for several miles, crossing a number of tributaries before it turns north after crossing Potter Run (6.1/1,356). From there, the trail continues north until it runs very close to I-80 (6.68/1,327). You won't be walking in untrammeled wilderness, but these several miles of trail are a vivid reminder of how precarious the existence of these last remaining stands of wilderness is. This section of the trail also offers views that—while not always beautiful, in the strict sense of the word—will certainly get your attention.

From the northernmost point of the trail near I-80, the AFT takes a hard right, climbs for a spell (about 700 feet), then winds away from civilization. The trail will eventually level out along an overgrown forest track and travel quietly along for several miles. A hunting lodge on the right signals that this section is ending (8.4/1,971). AFT swings left on the driveway to the lodge, cuts left through the forest, and then crosses Huckleberry Road. A sign there states that Shingle Mill Trail is just 0.5 mile ahead. That half-mile is passed on a moderately steep, switchbacked descent, but it won't be long before you reach the intersection with Shingle Mill Trail (on the right), as well as the trail register (9.0/1,720).

The AFT drops down to the lovely Black Moshannon Creek, which it follows for a few tenths of a mile through a thick forest of rhododendron. Keep your eye out for campsites on the right. The path eventually crosses the bridge at the foot of a hunting lodge (9.75/1,675). Look out for the trail behind the lodge on the right.

The trail continues upstream along Benner Run through an especially thick forest. Eventually, the trail climbs gradually and leaves the waterway behind; you'll see some orange blazes mixed in with the yellow. The trail drops down into and then follows Hall Run, crosses Tram Road (13.8/2,129), and then turns right as Forks Trail comes in from the left. You'll hike for a time following both blue and yellow blazes, with the middle branch of Rock Run below you on the left. The blue-blazed Rock Run Trail splits off from the AFT to the left and crosses the creek on a bridge (15.1/1,953). The AFT continues straight under yellow blazes, crossing a few creeks that form the headwaters of Benner Run.

You'll know you're nearing PA 504 when you pass a meadow and enter a grove of red spruce. Soon enough you'll see a telecommunications relay on your left, and then you'll reach the parking lot on PA 504 (18.6/2,368).

From the parking lot, the trail crosses directly across PA 504 and will soon descend fairly steeply down an old forest road. Do pay attention, however, as the footpath diverges quickly from the road to the right (18.9/2,105) and begins a steep and rocky, if short, climb to level terrain and partial views. Over the next several miles, the AFT follows the Allegheny Front with views to the south. This section is perhaps the most challenging, but it also offers the most rewarding views. After a steep descent along Whetstone Run (19.5/2,074), the AFT crosses a sidehill, then climbs for a vista. It will repeat this pattern a few times, eventually reaching Ralph's Pretty Good View (21.4/2,120) and Ralph's Majestic Vista (21.6/2,141).

From Ralph's Majestic Vista, the AFT turns west, climbs over a few rocky outcroppings (the "Stone Steps"), and then drops sharply down to Underwood Road (22.1/2,052), where the blazes will change to red. After about 1.5 miles of walking through fairly level forest, the trail will reach Smays Run and the campsite there (23.8/1,891).

Past Smays Run, walk about 1 mile on the red-blazed trail that takes you toward Julian Pike. If you follow the red-blazed trail faithfully, it will take you to the parking lot on Julian Pike—the blazes lead in, but they don't lead out

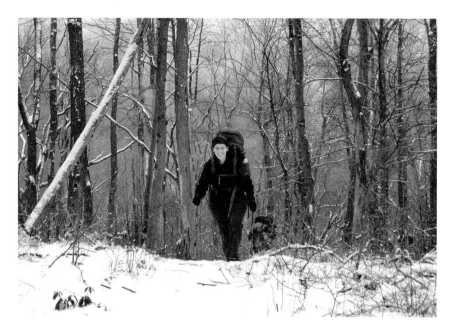

Two backpackers summit a crest on the Allegheny Front during a shoulder-season snowstorm.

again. Instead, look for a rightward bend that takes you across Julian Pike north of the parking lot. If you miss the bend (as I did), just walk north on the road for a few hundred yards and you'll eventually spot a sign marking the AFT, which changes back to yellow blazes here.

As the signs warn, the next section of trail is boggy as the path winds around the southern shore of Black Moshannon Lake. After about 2.5 miles, another potential snarl occurs: the trail continues northward on Moss-Hanne Trail (the companion trail to Shingle Mill Trail), or bends leftward as the AFT reaches for Shirks Road. Both trails are marked yellow (27.9/1,907). Just follow the sign and bend left. In short order, you'll reach Shirks Road, where you'll turn right, cross a bridge, pass a cabin, and turn left to follow Black Moshannon Creek (28.7/1,876).

While lovely, the southwestern quadrant of the trail is circuitous. It pays to be alert to the blazes, as they do shift color (orange, red, and yellow). Head southward with Black Moshannon Creek on your left. The terrain is often boggy, and there are a few well-constructed plank bridges. Eventually, the trail turns right, away from the creek, and crosses Clay Mine Road (30.4/1,972). The blazes turn red, and the trail drops and then climbs steadily to Wolf Rock Road (31.3/2,008). Take a left, follow the road uphill, and then, just before a gate, follow the blazes to cut off a corner of the road and begin descending (with orange blazes) on Beaver Road. You'll pass a bridge and have an opportunity to look up a long and dispiriting-looking climb along a road. Rejoice: the trail turns right and picks up the headwaters of Six Mile Run (32/1,907). The blazes are once again yellow.

After walking about 0.75 mile through an enchanting section of forest, the trail descends a bit and edges its way around Wolf Rocks. Cross Horse Hollow Road, pass a domicile, follow a tributary named Slide Run (34.0/1,850), and then begin a long but moderately graded climb (about 300 feet). The trail passes through a 2.5-mile section of forest before descending fairly steeply to Six Mile Run Road (36.6/1,808). Cross the river on a bridge, turn left on a footpath, and enjoy walking through a beautiful pine plantation of tall, straight evergreens.

The final section of trail is a bit of a detour. You'll have been following Six Mile Run for some time when the trail climbs up over the ridge on your right (37.4/1,820). When the AFT descends again, it follows a tributary of Six Mile Run to meet up with the main creek. Then the trail climbs, dips, and crosses sidehills for the final mile of the trip.

The path soon switchbacks down to PA 504. Cross the bridge to return to the parking lot (39.6/1,623).

OTHER OPTIONS

In the center of the AFT, Shingle Mill Trail and Moss-Hanne Trail cut across Black Moshannon State Park, facilitating a number of different options.

Instead of hiking the entire trail in one trip, you could use the connector trails to hike the eastern and western loops over the course of two weekends. This would be a fine project for beginner or intermediate backpackers looking to extend their ranges—the western loop adds up to about 31 miles and the eastern loop about 30 miles. Both loops are charming, and neither is especially difficult. You could use the parking lots on Six Mile Run, Julian Pike, or the one in the center of the park to orchestrate such a trip.

Few options are available for extending the trip, but of course one could always decrease the AFT's difficulty by slowing down and covering fewer miles per day over a longer period of time. There are three other trailhead parking lots that would facilitate variants: the parking lot for the state park in the center of the trail; the parking lot for the AFT on the far eastern side of the loop, near the Allegheny Front itself; and the southeasterly parking lot on Julian Pike.

NEARBY

The town of Philipsburg, Pennsylvania, is just a few miles west of the trailhead on PA 504 and offers an assortment of restaurants, gas stations, motels, and services. Also, State College is just a few miles away, with all the pubs and restaurants you'd expect of a college town its size.

ADDITIONAL INFORMATION

Contact the Pennsylvania Department of Conservation and Natural Resources at 814-765-0821 for additional information and the latest printed map of the AFT. Black Moshannon State Park (814-342-5960) is also a good resource for learning about the area.

TRIP 17
CALEDONIA DREAMING

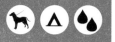

Location: Caledonia State Park and Michaux State Forest, Pennsylvania

Highlights: Secluded Hozack Hollow, a rare lakeside walk around Long Pine Run Reservoir, and views of Rocky Knob

Distance: 19.6 miles round-trip

Total Elevation Gain/Loss: 3,379 feet gain/3,379 feet loss

Trip Length: 2–3 days

Difficulty: Moderate

Recommended Maps and Other Resources:

- Potomac Appalachian Trail Club, *Map 2-3, Appalachian Trail, PA Route 94 to US Route 30,* 2013. dcnr.state.pa.us/cs/groups/public/ documents/document/dcnr_004834.pdf.
- Appalachian Mountain Club, *Pennsylvania Highlands Regional Recreational Map and Guide.*
- USGS Quad: Caledonia Park.

A gentle trip suitable for new backpackers, this "lollipop loop" will take you high up the Pennsylvania Blue Ridge, along a memorable lakeshore, and up and over Rocky Knob. It will also give you a taste of the close Pennsylvania hollows, with their thickets of rhododendron and mountain laurel. You'll end the trip with 9 miles of walking on the Appalachian Trail (AT) southbound into Caledonia State Park.

HIKE OVERVIEW

From Caledonia State Park, walk northbound on the AT, but quickly diverge to follow a number of side trails—Hozack Hollow, Greenwood, Beaver, and Rocky Knob trails—to make a loop that joins up with the AT just south of Shippensburg Road. From there, enjoy the AT's relatively level path southbound as it follows the ridgeline, eventually retracing the route you walked in on near Quarry Gap Shelter.

Appalachian Mountain Club (AMC) and partner organizations, including the National Park Service Rivers, Trails, and Conservation Assistance Program (RTCA), have included Caledonia State Park and Michaux State Forest in their collaborative plan to create a trail network in the region. The Pennsylvania

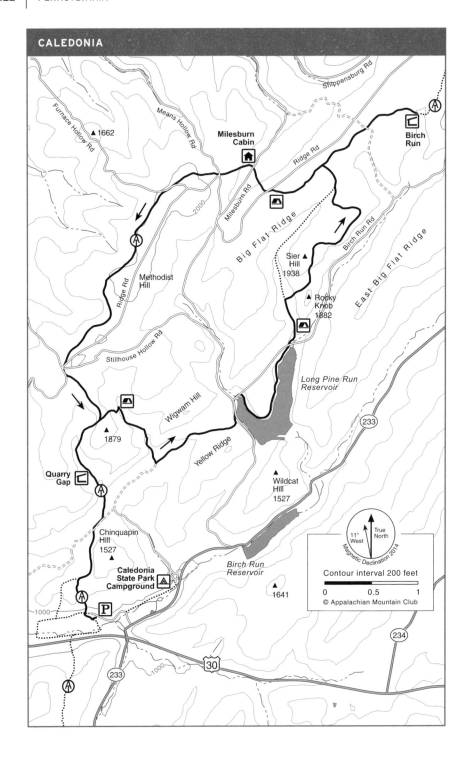

CALEDONIA

Highlands Trail Network would not only extend the existing Highlands Trail from the Delaware River to the Maryland border, but would also connect major existing trail systems in the state—including the AT. For more information, visit highlandsmobile.outdoors.org and hikethehighlands.outdoors.org.

HOW TO REACH THE TRAILHEAD

From where I-81 passes through Chambersburg, Pennsylvania, take US 30 east about 8.5 miles. You'll see signs for the AT as you near the park. Turn left onto PA 233, and then take another quick left into Caledonia State Park and drive to a parking lot, toward the back, where there is a restroom. You should be able to spot the white blazes of the AT as the trail passes nearby (39° 54.5621' N, 77° 29.0584' W).

OVERNIGHT OPTIONS

You'll have a wide variety of places to spend the night on this loop. Both of the AT shelters are attractive destinations; however, the AT does see a lot of traffic along this section. You'll enjoy a more secluded experience by camping along Knob Run or Hozack Run, which are ideal backcountry sites.

Camping is allowed throughout Michaux State Forest without a permit so long as you stay only one night. If you stay multiple nights at a single site, then you will need to request a free permit. Your campsite has to be at least 25 feet from a trail and at least 100 feet from a stream.

Quarry Gap Shelter (1.95/1,436/39° 55.919' N, 77° 29.183' W). About 2 miles into the loop, this is one of the prettiest, best maintained trail shelters along the AT. Quarry Gap Shelter has excellent access to water, a privy, and tent pads nearby.

Hozack Run (3.0/1,583/39° 56.463' N, 77° 28.753' W). Once you turn east of the AT, you'll quickly descend into the beautiful hollow cut by Hozack Run. After a few switchbacks, you'll come upon a campsite just as the trail reaches the bottom of the hollow.

Knob Run (6.7/1,407/39° 57.152' N, 77° 26.654' W). With Long Pine Run Reservoir behind you, you'll begin walking northward on Rocky Knob Trail. Just as you pass the road, there are several tent sites with easy access to water.

Birch Run Shelter (10.5/1,794/39° 59.107' N, 77° 25.166' W). Just south of Shippensburg Road, you'll reach this AT shelter with numerous tent sites nearby. It can be a crowded spot, so come early if you're planning to stay. Water is nearby.

Milesburn Road (12.4/1,917/39° 58.392' N, 77° 26.862' W). As you're headed south on the AT toward Milesburn Road, you'll be walking along a broad ridge with plenty of flat ground under sheltering pines. Just before the little descent into Milesburn Road, you'll spot a broad primitive site on the left.

If you're interested in more luxurious overnight accommodations, Caledonia State Park offers vehicle camping, and PATC's Milesburn Cabin is also on this route.

HIKE DESCRIPTION

From the parking lot, begin following the white-blazed AT north as it meanders through the last few hundred yards of the developed picnic area. The trail crosses a road, then takes you up a stout little climb of about 400 feet before it levels out on the shoulder of Chinquapin Hill (1,552). Pass an intersection with Three Valley Trail on your left (0.5/1,280), then walk very briefly on Greenwood Furnace Road. Bear left and continue following the AT. Climb through a tunnel of rhododendron, then arrive at Quarry Gap Shelter, an excellent spot for a break (2.0/1,451).

You'll find rocky footing as you head north from the shelter, crossing a creek over a small log bridge. Climb gently for about 400 feet, but keep your eyes open for blue-blazed Hozack Hollow Trail on the right (2.7/1,818). Here, turn right, leave the AT, and drop down via a series of switchbacks to an idyllic little run (3.0/1,583). The trail winds its way through this valley, occasionally passing over the run, though the crossings are easily rock-hoppable.

When Hozack Hollow Trail meets Greenwood Trail (3.83/1,282), turn left onto this broad old road grade that climbs, then gently descends to Milesburn Road (4.96/1,379). This trail is blazed blue until a power line, and then is blazed red. You'll see the waters of Long Pine Run Reservoir through the trees. Turn left onto the road, then swing a quick right onto Birch Run Road. The road crosses a creek on a bridge; look out for yellow-blazed Beaver Trail to the right (5.22/1,371). This trail follows the shores of the reservoir, going first to a small beach, then heading northward along the water's edge. You won't find many opportunities to stroll along a lakeshore in the Mid-Atlantic.

When the trail climbs back up to Birch Run Road, put the lake behind you (6.5/1,398). For the next 2.75 miles, follow Rocky Knob Trail (blazed orange), which at first crosses, and then follows, a creek bottom. This trail is a bit of a curiosity, as it soon splits (7.06/1,507), with the leftward branch climbing up the run and the rightward branch ascending about 200 feet to a saddle beneath Rocky Knob (1,872), the hill that stands out above the north end of the reservoir. Both arrive in the same place, but you should take the rightward branch. Past the saddle, the trail ascends Sier Hill (7.64/1,930) and follows the ridgeline for a ways. Look back for a view of the reservoir.

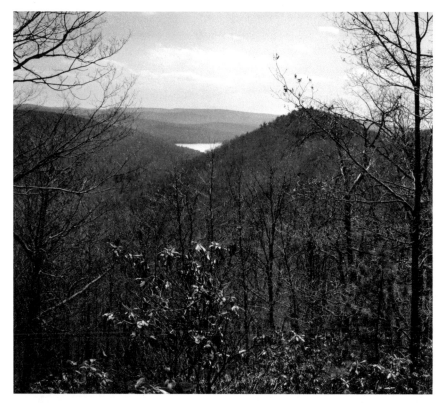

Past Rocky Knob, you'll be able to peer over the knob's shoulder to catch a glimpse of Long Pine Run Reservoir.

Soon, the trail turns eastward, reunites with its leftward branch, and rejoins the AT (9.19/1,899). If you turn north, you'll have a little more than 1 mile of easy walking before you reach Birch Run Shelter, which boasts an excellent spring and, of course, good spots for tenting (10.5/1,796).

From Birch Run Shelter, 9 miles of walking southbound along the AT will complete the loop. After the intersection of Rocky Knob Trail and the AT, continue south along a broad, flat ridge. Eventually, the AT crosses Ridge Road and then descends to Milesburn Hollow, where the Potomac Appalachian Trail Club owns a cabin (12.8/1,683). Climb from this creek to regain the ridge and pass another road intersection (13.2/1,961). Do pay careful attention at these intersections; the AT is well marked, but it is possible to lose the trail as you cross. Always make sure you have a blaze.

For the next 3 miles, walk on the western side of Big Flat Ridge with its obscured views of pastoral countryside to the west. The AT crosses Haunted Hollow Road and traverses a complicated intersection where a number of roads meet. Here, turn left briefly onto one of the roads for a few hundred feet before the trail regains the forest on the left (16.3/1,988). The AT turns east and begins a 500-foot descent toward Quarry Gap. Soon, you'll be on familiar ground, including the Quarry Gap Shelter (17.7/1,451). Two miles of continued downhill walking will return you to your vehicle at Caledonia State Park (19.6/928).

OTHER OPTIONS

Because this loop is rather self-contained, you have limited options for lengthening or shortening it. You can always add distance by parking your vehicle farther north or south along the AT and walking out-and-back miles before starting this loop. If you walk very far south, you can link up with the Maryland AT hikes described in this book—Pen-Mar is only about 18 miles south of Caledonia State Park.

NEARBY

With Gettysburg, Pennsylvania, just few additional miles east along US 30, you can find an array of restaurants and businesses catering to tourists. On a day when the weather is fine, few things can top a post-hike lunch on Gettysburg's town circle.

ADDITIONAL INFORMATION

Visit Michaux State Forest online at dcnr.state.pa.us/forestry/stateforests/michaux/ or call 717-352-2211 and Caledonia State Park online at dcnr.state.pa.us/stateparks/findapark/caledonia/ for more information.

TRIP 18
WELCOME TO THE FOREST PRIMEVAL

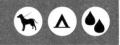

Location: Susquehannock State Forest, Pennsylvania
Highlights: Lush, verdant forests; immaculate seclusion; and the ultimate sustained Allegheny Plateau hiking experience
Distance: 81 miles round-trip
Total Elevation Gain/Loss: 13,050 feet gain/13,050 feet loss
Trip Length: 4–10 days
Difficulty: Epic
Recommended Maps and Other Resources:
- Chuck Dillon, *A Guide to the Susquehannock Trail System*. Wellsboro, PA: Pine Creek Press, 1997.
- Susquehannock Trail Club. *Trail Maps* (stc-hike.org/Gear.php).
- USGS Quads: Brookland, Cherry Springs, Oleona, Young Womans Creek, Tamarack, Short Run, Conrad, and Ayers Hill.

Almost all of Potter County, Pennsylvania, was clear-cut in the late nineteenth and early twentieth centuries, but the second-growth forest surrounding the Susquehannock Trail System (STS) will take your breath away with its lush growth, woodland variety, unrelenting beauty, and abundance of wildlife. Leave the workaday world far behind and ramble along some of the most isolated territory in the Mid-Atlantic, whether you're out for a week or a long weekend.

HIKE OVERVIEW

Founded in the late 1960s, when Bill Fish and other members of the Susquehannock Trail Club decided to weave together numerous trails in the region to form a loop that would support an immersive wilderness experience, the STS is one of the elder statesmen of Pennsylvania's long-distance backpacking trails. Starting at the north portal near Denton, this route takes you on a clockwise loop around the region, passing by Lyman Run State Park and Ole Bull State Park before arriving at the village of Cross Fork. You'll return north through the Hammersley Wild Area—one of the largest wildernesses in the state and a haven for wildlife.

Hiking along the STS ranges from quite easy to fairly strenuous. Section-hiking this trip is certainly possible (see Other Options), but you'll want to

SUSQUEHANNOCK NORTH

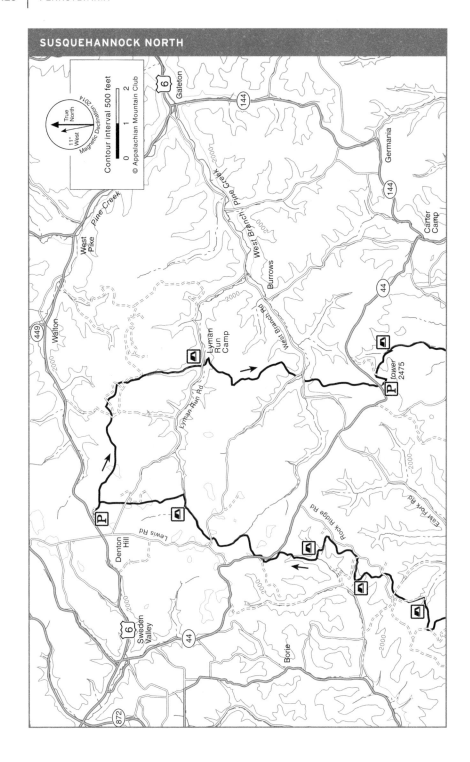

SUSQUEHANNOCK SOUTH

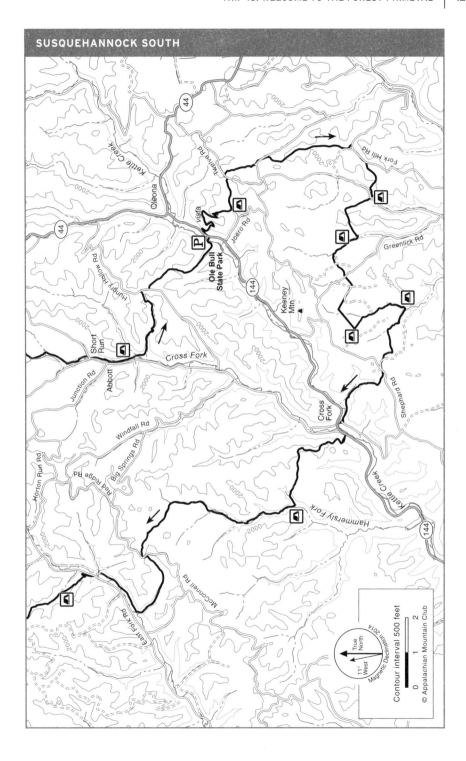

Contour interval 500 feet

0   1   2

© Appalachian Mountain Club

True North

11° West

Magnetic Declination 2014

be an experienced and fit backpacker before you thru-hike this Pennsylvania classic in its entirety.

HOW TO REACH THE TRAILHEAD

From Williamsport, Pennsylvania, head north on US 15 and drive about 27 miles toward Mansfield. Take the exit for PA 414 and head west. Drive about 10 miles until you reach the little town of Morris. Bear right onto PA 287, and drive north 10 miles until you reach Wellsboro. Take a left onto Main Street, which becomes PA 660 and then PA 362 as it continues west toward Ansonia. When you reach Ansonia, take a left onto US 6. About 26 miles later, after you pass Ski Denton on your left, you'll take a left onto the road for the Susquehannock State Forest District Office. Park in the gravel parking lot on the right (41° 46.106′ N, 77° 52.177′ W).

OVERNIGHT OPTIONS

Backcountry, primitive camping is allowed in the state forest and does not require a permit if you are staying for just one night. You may, however, want to keep your group fairly small: there are few sites that will accommodate more than a couple of tents.

Lyman Run (7/1,671/41° 43.262′ N, 77° 47.169′ W). One of the better campsites on the trail is located just past the bridge that crosses Lyman Run.

Hogback Hollow (15.3/1,758/41° 38.530′ N, 77° 46.677′ W). Once you've passed PA 44 and the Cherry Springs Fire Tower, the trail descends steeply into Hogback Hollow, where there are several smallish campsites on the left.

Short Run (20.6/1,327/41° 34.342′ N, 77° 46.932′ W). When the trail enters the flat river bottom where Short Run, Yochum Run, Cherry Run, and Dry Hollow drain into Cross Fork, look for a number of well-placed campsites suitable for larger groups. Most of the hunting camps in this area are on private land. Request permission if you want to camp in the fields near the cabins.

Ole Bull State Park (26.1/1,210/41° 32.358′ N, 77° 42.954′ W). If you'd like to stay in an established campground, you may pay a small fee and do so at this attractive park, though your tent will likely be dwarfed by the RVs.

Impson Hollow (29.1/1,445/41° 31.739′ N, 77° 41.943′ W). From Ole Bull State Park, the trail switchbacks up to the plateau and then quickly drops down to this hollow, where there are two hunters' cabins. A grassy margin offers reasonable camping with easy access to water.

Morgan Hollow (36.2/1,326/41° 28.153′ N, 77° 41.550′ W). After the exceptionally steep descent down this hollow, the trail reaches Young Womans Creek, where there is a good-sized campsite.

Scoval Branch (41.4/1,610/41° 28.592′ N, 77° 45.909′ W). Once you leave the pipeline cut, the trail follows Scoval Branch for about 2 miles. You'll find several small tent sites along this creek, including one right where the trail leaves the cut.

Hammersley Wild Area (52.1/1,260/41° 30.148′ N, 77° 51.800′ W). Past the village of Cross Fork, the STS climbs up and over the plateau and then drops down to Hammersley Wild Area. Numerous campsites may be found along Hammersley Fork. The site where the trail first meets the creek is especially beautiful.

Stony Run (63.5/1,615/41° 36.137′ N, 77° 54.666′ W). Once you leave Sinnemahoning Creek, the STS starts a series of fairly steep climbs and descents. Camping at Stony Run—a small campsite in a beautiful, fern-robed gully—will enable you to break up this section. Similar sites are available at Wild Boy Hollow (66.6/1,877) and the intersection of Prouty Place Trail (69.5/1,723).

Ford Hollow (72/1,773/41° 40.349′ N, 77° 53.469′ W). About 2 miles south of Patterson Park, the STS drops down into Hockney Hollow, turns right across the mountain, and takes a left on a road grade to reach this grassy area alongside the creek, where a good-sized group may camp. Note that the large meadow farther along is private land.

Splash Dam Hollow (77.6/2,015/41° 43.770′ N, 77° 51.938′ W). While you're just 3.5 miles away from the northern portal, this is an attractive campsite that will accommodate several tents.

HIKE DESCRIPTION

From the parking lot, walk in toward the trail on a gravel road that serves the outbuildings of the district forestry office. As the road bends left, follow the trail uphill slightly to the right as it becomes a footpath. The trail register and the orange blazes of the STS await (0.58/2,454). Sign in, and begin walking to the left to follow the trail clockwise. Over the next 7 miles, you'll enjoy easy walking as the path at first stays up high on the plateau and then begins a gentle descent along Jacobs Hollow to Lyman Run. As you walk through this lush forest with its undergrowth of ferns, you'll pass a vista to your left (2.81/2.436), then cross Thompson Road (3.26/2,266) and Ridge Road (4.54/2,214). The trail then heads downhill more seriously on the left bank of the creek. When it crosses to the right, you'll know that you've almost reached the road leading to Lyman Run State Park (6.9/1,698). Beyond it, a suspension footbridge takes you over the stream and to the campsite there (7/1,671).

Next, the STS climbs about 600 feet to regain the plateau (8.43/2,293), where you'll enjoy level ground for about 2 miles. The trail then descends to meet Sunken Branch and the West Branch of Pine Creek. As you leave the forest, take a left on the gravel road, then a hard right on the paved West Branch Road (11/1,670). The path follows this road briefly, but then takes a left that almost seems to climb through the front lawn of a nearby house (11.2/1,706). This is Cardiac Climb, which gains 700 feet over the next 0.9 mile—one of the trip's tougher challenges.

From the plateau's top (12.1/2,363), more easy miles follow until you cross PA 44 and pass the Cherry Springs Fire Tower (13.6/2,456). The trail drops down to a trail register, crosses an abandoned railroad grade next to a cabin, and then enters Hogback Hollow. For several miles, the STS stays on the right above the stream—you'll spot a few beaver dams—but then settles down to follow some road grades as it reaches the flat stream bottom of Cross Fork Creek. At about mile 19, the trail bends abruptly to the left, then to the right, and reaches Short Run Road (19.2/1,408). It turns right on this road briefly, but then hangs left just before a bridge leading to Boone Road (19.3/1,390). Continue along this stream for 1.2 miles more before crossing Yochum Run on a bridge (20.5/1,325).

A climb along Cherry Run brings you to Hungry Hollow Road (23.3/2,072). The STS turns right, continues about 0.2 mile on the road, then branches off to the left, reentering the forest. After about 0.8 mile on the plateau, the path begins a 2-mile descent into Ole Bull State Park along Ole Bull Run—both are named after a Norwegian violinist who founded a short-lived colony here in 1844. The STS's route through this pretty little park passes over a bridge spanning Kettle Creek and a bathroom with trashcans (26.1/1,210).

Immediately on leaving the park, the STS crosses PA 144 and begins a stout, switchbacked climb of about 1,000 feet back up to the plateau—a view allows you to glimpse the ruggedness of this country. Quickly, though, the trail follows a stream down into Impson Hollow, where it crosses a run in a grassy area between two hunting lodges (29.1/1,445). A gentle climb, at first along a road grade, delivers you to Twelve Mile Road (30/1,948). Take a left to walk along it for 0.25 mile, then regain the forest to your right. A sign for Spook Hollow will caution you about "proper" behavior in this area. I've passed through twice, and the phantoms haven't barred my passage … yet.

With any luck, you'll emerge unscathed from this terrifying place. The STS then passes an intersection for North Link Trail—which connects to Black Forest Trail (Trip 15)—meanders around the cabins on Big Spring Branch, and traverses southward for several miles through rich forestlands. After pass-

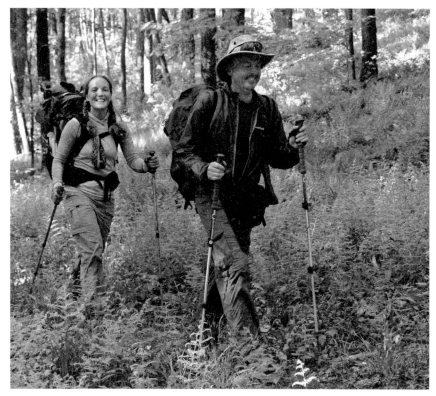

Hikers enjoy a stroll through the verdant forests of the Allegheny Plateau in north-central Pennsylvania.

ing through some game gates and by the intersection for South Link Trail (also leading to the Black Forest Trail), the STS arrives at Fork Hill Road (34.2/2,078). Take a right and follow this road for 0.75 mile. A sign marks where Donut Hole Trail comes up from the south. The STS, which here takes a sharp right into the forest (35/2,069), shares footway with this 90-mile trail for the next 8.1 miles. The blazes remain orange, but you may see some red paint too.

Soon, the STS plunges precipitously down Morgan Hollow, a rocky and treacherous descent that ends with a bridge (Ted's Truss) over Young Woman's Creek (36.2/1,389). A climb up the seldom walked Long Hollow follows, with the trail immediately dipping down Bobsled Hollow to turn right along Greenlick Run (37.9/1,462). As you follow this beautiful stream on fragments of an old logging railroad grade, the countryside opens out and you'll need to keep a sharp eye out for blazes. Eventually, the trail takes a left to climb up over a low hill and down Italian Hollow (38.8/1,541).

In this area, the terrain is more open and the STS passes several wells, follows a road, and finally takes a left onto a pipeline cut, which affords you a rare glimpse of unobstructed sky. You'll walk down, up, and down this cut before the trail exits left and begins following the brushy left bank of Scoval Branch (41.4/1,610). Just under 2 miles later, Donut Hole Trail heads downstream on Shingle Branch (43.1/1,451) while the STS turns northwest up Porter Branch to make for Cross Fork. A climb up Green Timber Hollow brings you to Culver Woods Road (45.3/1,847), which you'll walk along for a bit before the trail crosses Shepard Road and begins a long, gentle, winding descent into town (47.6/1,004).

After a well-earned break in civilization, cross the Main Street bridge over Kettle Creek and turn left on PA 144, which you'll follow for about 0.5 mile before the trail leaves the road to the right (48.4/1,113) and immediately makes for the plateau via a steady climb. The path remains up high for almost 2 miles before it drops down via a hollow into Hammersley Fork Valley—the largest area without a road in Pennsylvania. After you take a right along Hammersley Fork Creek (52/1,252), pass a trail register and begin about 8 miles of walking through this beautiful and secluded wilderness, first on the east bank of the creek, then on the west.

The STS passes the popular swimming hole known as Hammersley Pool, then begins a very gentle climb north. The grade steepens somewhat just before you reach McConnell Road (58.1/1,987), but quickly relents and treats you to an easy walk down to Sinnemahoning Creek. The STS takes a right here (60.3/1,317) and follows a road through this picturesque river valley. The blazes are few and far between, but continue to follow the road until it crosses the creek on a dilapidated bridge (another great swimming hole!) and turns right on East Fork Road (62.2/1,380), which it briefly follows before reaching another trail register in the frontyard of a farmhouse.

With their quick succession of ascents and descents, the next 10 miles are perhaps the hardest of the route. From East Fork Road, the trail first climbs steeply about 600 feet, flirting with a road grade that it eventually settles on as it slides down to meet Stony Run (63.5/1,615). You then face a steady climb of 2.3 miles and 700 feet up a close Pennsylvania hollow before the trail tops out (65.6/2,369), passes by the remains of the Old Stove, and then drops down along an old road grade to Wild Boy Run (66.6/1,877). The path climbs for the plateau again, then takes an especially steep, straight descent down to Prouty Place Trail (69.5/1,723). After one more climb, walk along the plateau's edge for a spell before yet another steep drop takes you down Hockney Hollow.

Toward the bottom, the trail darts right over the foot of the mountain and reaches a grassy road grade in Ford Hollow (72/1,773).

With this stretch of trail behind you, the last 9 miles of the STS will seem relaxing. From Ford Hollow, the trail ascends gently on an old grassy road. The trail then turns right (73/1,921), becomes more of a footpath, and then parallels PA 44 as it approaches Patterson Park. You'll cross the road there (74.2/2,482) and walk down a grassy grade to reach the West Branch of Pine Creek (75/2,171). A brief climb takes you across Sunken Branch Road (76.4/2,469), then the trail descends and follows Splash Dam Hollow for about 1.5 miles. A sharp left-hand turn (78/2,043) will take you up your final climb, as you regain the plateau at the trail's highest point of 2,531 feet (79.3). A little more easy walking leads you back to the first trail register and the beginning of the loop (80.5/2,450). After a sharp left, you'll be back to your vehicle (81/2,406).

OTHER OPTIONS

While it's unlikely you'll want to add miles to this already demanding loop, the STS shares its path for about 8.1 miles with 90-mile Donut Hole Trail, and North and South Link trails will take you to Black Forest Trail. A backpacker with ample free time could ramble about for weeks on the Allegheny Plateau.

More relevantly, you may want to section-hike the STS so that you can complete it in more manageable segments. You could divide it into a segment from Denton Hill to Ole Bull State Park (26.5 miles), a second segment from Ole Bull to Cross Fork (23 miles), and a third section from Cross Fork back to Denton Hill (34.5 miles).

NEARBY

Of course, the STS passes through the little town of Cross Fork, Pennsylvania, where there are several businesses catering to anglers, hunters, and hikers. The nearest good-sized towns are Coudersport and Wellsboro, Pennsylvania, and Wellsville and Olean, New York. Williamsport is the gateway to the region—it features all the services you might require.

ADDITIONAL INFORMATION

For more information on the STS, contact the Susquehannock District Office of the Pennsylvania Department of Conservation and Natural Resources at dcnr.state.pa.us/forestry/stateforests/susquehannock/ or 814-274-3600. The STS is maintained by the Susquehannock Trail Club, which can be found at stc-hike.org. The club offers a patch for those who complete the trail, whether they do so by thru-hiking or section-hiking.

4

NEW YORK

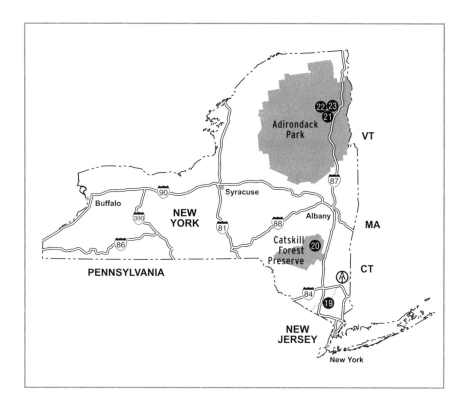

TRIP 19
CENTRAL PARK

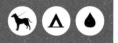

Location: Harriman State Park, New York

Highlights: Bear Mountain, views of the Hudson and New York City, West Mountain

Distance: 11.4 miles round-trip

Total Elevation Gain/Loss: 3,242 feet of gain/3,242 feet of loss

Trip Length: 2 days

Difficulty: Moderate

Recommended Maps and Other Resources:

- *Northern Harriman Bear Mountain Trails.* Trail Map 119. 14th ed. New York–New Jersey Trail Conference, 2012.
- USGS Quads: Popolopen Lake, and Peekskill.

Marvel at how wild and secluded Harriman State Park feels, with almost 50,000 acres of forestland, all within an hour of New York City. Backpackers will find nearly limitless opportunities to explore and perfect their backcountry craft in this expansive and beautiful park.

HIKE OVERVIEW

From the Anthony Wayne Recreation Area on the Palisades, this route takes you up onto the ridgeline of West Mountain, where you'll enjoy views of the park, Hudson River, and Bear Mountain before reaching a shelter that offers a splendid southward vista. On a clear evening, New York City can just be made out on the horizon. The next morning, you'll journey through the deep and surprisingly secluded forests of the park before regaining the Appalachian Trail (AT) at Hessian Lake and tackling the climb up to Bear Mountain itself, where spectacular views await.

HOW TO REACH THE TRAILHEAD

From New York City, head north on the Palisades Interstate Parkway. Just before you reach US 6, take Exit 17 for the Anthony Wayne Recreation Area, where you'll find a very large parking area (41° 17.8012' N, 74° 1.6667' W).

Most other backpackers will be approaching on I-87. Take Exit 16 and follow signs for NY 17/US 6/Harriman. Pay your toll and take a left onto NY 17, then another left on US 6, which you'll follow for about 6.4 miles into the

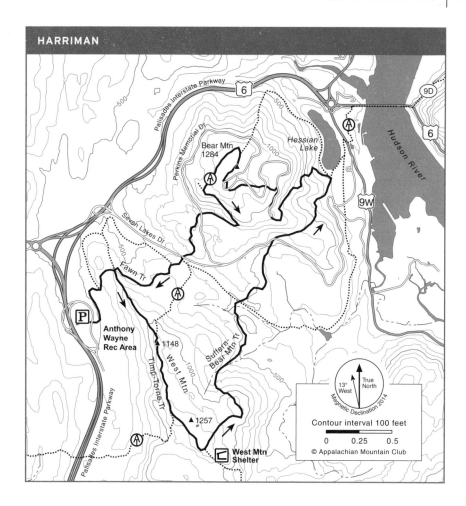

park. At the traffic circle, take the second exit and merge onto the Palisades Interstate Parkway South. Then, take Exit 17 and follow the directions above.

OVERNIGHT OPTIONS

Backcountry camping is allowed in Harriman State Park only at established campsites or at designated shelters, which are available on a first-come, first-served basis. If a shelter is occupied when you arrive, you may camp within 300 feet. You'll spot plenty of tent sites in the vicinity. Campfires are allowed only in the fireplaces at the shelters.

West Mountain Shelter (2.7/1,194/41° 16.947' N, 74° 00.564' W). After you leave the AT, you'll walk about 0.5 mile southward, pass a yellow-blazed trail to the north, and then come upon this ideally situated shelter. On a clear night, you'll enjoy a view of the Hudson River and possibly the towers of Manhattan away in the south. There is no water at this shelter, so you'll need to carry in your water.

Given the restrictions on camping, this trip is best hiked as a weekend overnighter, with the night passed at this shelter.

HIKE DESCRIPTION

From the parking lot, it can be a bit tricky to get started hiking on the trail system. Walk toward the recreation area proper, and take a left to pass a field used for picnics and a building with restrooms. Take a right on the white-blazed trail (0.5/513), which climbs gently up to meet Beechy Bottom Road on the left, while Fawn Trail (red-blazed on white) heads straight uphill into the forest (0.6/522/41° 18.033' N, 74° 01.534' W).

Follow Fawn Trail briefly, climbing up to meet blue-blazed Timp-Torne Trail in a saddle atop West Mountain (0.8/695). Follow the blue blazes to the right and to climb over rocky slabs. The rewards are immediate, as there are a number of excellent views, both of the park to the west (looking back over the Palisades) and of Bear Mountain and the Hudson River to the east (1.1/941). You'll want take this climb slowly, savoring each of these spots.

Soon the AT joins the route from your left (that way lies Maine; 1.4/1,097) and the trails continue together along the ridgeline of West Mountain. The trails climb up and down along this ridgeline. A few scrambly sections will test you, then the AT will head off to your right (that way lies Georgia; 2.06/1,189). Continue to follow the blue blazes along the mountaintop until you reach yellow-blazed Suffern-Bear Mountain Trail, which comes in from the right (2.29/1,207) and, a little later, leaves to the left (2.5/1,217). Take note: this will be your route for tomorrow. For now, follow Timp-Torne Trail past its intersection with northbound Suffern-Bear Mountain Trail and quickly reach the West Mountain Shelter about 0.2 miles later (2.7/1,194), where you'll find more great views.

The next morning, return to the yellow blazes and take a right to head north on the Suffern-Bear Mountain Trail (2.9/1,217). It will drop down briefly, climb a bit, and then start a long and somewhat steep descent before it reaches a creek (3.9/637). Refill your bottles, cross, and follow the trail as it crosses, first, the Bridle Path of deserted Revolutionary War-era Doodletown, and then the 1777 ski trail. The trail ascends, crosses Seven Lakes Drive (5.2/542), and then climbs over the shoulder of Bear Mountain before dropping down to Hessian Lake.

Follow the trail to the shore of the lake, where you should be able to locate the white blazes of the AT as it rounds the lake's south side (6.0/178). Take a left

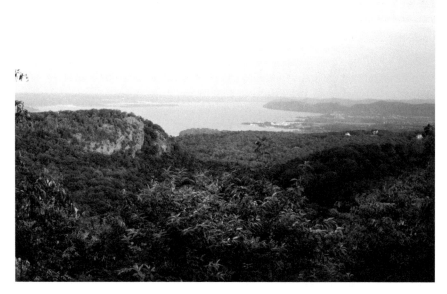

From near the West Mountain Shelter in Harriman State Park, you'll enjoy views of the Hudson River.

and head west, or southbound, on the AT. The trail quickly begins a sustained climb of more than 1,000 feet up Bear Mountain. A great deal of work has been done on this section of trail so that it can handle the crowds of people who visit each year. The first 0.8 mile of the climb takes place on beautiful rock staircases. At present, however, this new trail is incomplete. Until it is finished, the trail turns right on Perkins Memorial Drive (6.87/908), follows it for a bit, then turns left to climb again through the woods on an ordinary footpath (7.13/997). The AT crosses the road two more times before it reaches the summit of Bear Mountain (7.75/1,284/41° 18.6389' N, 74° 0.3917' W). Take in the views of the Hudson River Valley, climb Perkins Tower, and learn about the history of the park from the exhibit inside the tower.

When you're ready to leave, follow the AT past the tower. It leads you across the flat summit of Bear Mountain, bringing you to one last view (8.13/1,267) before cutting sharply and beginning a steady 600-foot descent down the mountain. The AT follows an old forest road for a spell, crosses Perkins Memorial Drive (9.34/778), and then crosses Seven Lakes Drive (9.8/607). Follow the AT through the forest until it intersects with red-blazed Fawn Trail (10.4/698). Take that right, pass blue-blazed Timp-Torne Trail, and arrive back at the white blazes of Anthony Wayne Trail (10.9/541). Retrace your steps to the picnic area and your waiting vehicle (11.4/476).

OTHER OPTIONS

Despite its proximity to Gotham, Harriman is a large, wild, and at times secluded-feeling park. Well worth exploring beyond the short loop presented here, a backpacker new to the pastime could certainly cut his or her teeth by wandering about, perhaps focusing on the AT, Long Path, and Suffern Mountain Trail. The Egg, in the southern half of the park, boasts quite a splendid view of the metropolis. Do be warned, however, that many of the trails are not as well maintained as the major arteries like the AT. Be prepared for route-finding issues, and always bring your map and compass.

NEARBY

You're a mere 30 miles away from the largest metropolis in the United States, so civilization is not far. There are also plenty of businesses clustered near I-87 Exit 16 in Harriman, New York.

ADDITIONAL INFORMATION

For additional information on Harriman State Park, visit the website maintained by the New York State Office of Parks, Recreation, and Historic Preservation at nysparks.com/parks/145. In case of emergency, call the New York State Park Police at 845-786-2781.

TRIP 20
A SEASON IN HELL

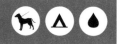

Location: Catskill Forest Preserve, New York

Highlights: Five peaks above 3,500 feet, endless views of the Catskills, Diamond Notch Falls, eternal bragging rights

Distance: 22.2 miles one-way

Total Elevation Gain/Loss: 8,686 feet gain/8,916 feet loss

Trip Length: 2–3 days

Difficulty: Strenuous

Recommended Maps and Other Resources:

- *Catskill Forest Preserve: Northeastern Catskill Trails.* New York–New Jersey Trail Conference. Trail Map 141. 9th edition. 2010.
- USGS Quads: Lexington, Hunter, Bearsville, Woodstock, and Kaaterskill.

You may not abandon hope, but you may find yourself wondering at your fate as you pass through the hiking gauntlet known as the Devil's Path. Early settlers of the region believed that the Devil built these mountains so that only he could scale them. You probably won't encounter Lucifer on your walk but, as you chase the Devil's Path up and down its home turf, you may wonder if the settlers might have been onto something. If you vanquish this devil of a trail, you'll be boasting about it the rest of your life.

HIKE OVERVIEW

If you're looking for bragging rights, the east-to-west jaunt along the Devil's Path will not disappoint. It's true: the farther west you go, the higher the Catskill Mountains get as the gaps between them get lower. Often cited as one of the toughest trails in the east, or even in the lower 48, this torturous path over several of the highest peaks in the Catskills will test the will of even the strongest backpackers. You may conclude that the archfiend did indeed have a hand in laying out its course.

Many Mid-Atlantic hikers tell horror stories of attempts to complete this trail, from hail storms, ice, and excruciating heat, to hikers left torn and bloody from the often steep, always rocky, sometimes unstable path. The terrain is unforgivingly vertical, either climbing straight up steeply or dropping down equally steeply in ways that may test your nerve. Flat ground is rare. Water is

DEVIL'S PATH

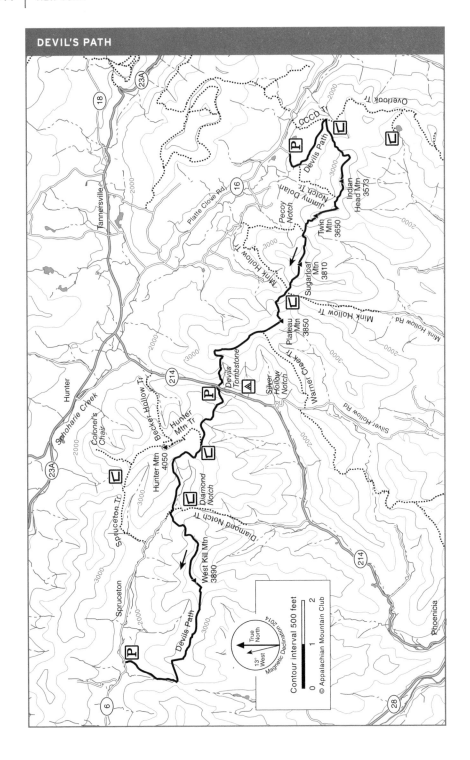

Contour interval 500 feet

True North

13° West

Magnetic Declination 2014

© Appalachian Mountain Club

0   1   2

scarce. And you can expect to do a scrambling move or two on many of the ascents and descents.

But the diabolical difficulty is balanced by the deliciously tempting challenge, as well as some of the best views of the rugged Catskills. And if you're looking to bag peaks in the Catskills, this route takes you over five of the official 35 peaks over 3,500 feet (Indian Head, Sugarloaf, Twin, Plateau, and West Kill) and within spitting distance of a sixth, Hunter Mountain. Fortunately, Devil's Path is quite well marked, so you won't have to worry about navigation, at least.

HOW TO REACH THE TRAILHEAD

To Reach the Ending Trailhead. Take Exit 19 off I-87, about halfway between New York City and Albany, and head west on NY 28. About 28 miles later, take a right on NY 42 and continue north for about 7 miles. Then, turn right on CR 6/Spruceton Road. Look for the parking bay on the right in about 3.8 miles (42° 11.5285' N, 74° 19.484' W).

To Reach the Starting Trailhead. From the eastern trailhead, return to NY 42 and turn to continue north about 4 miles. Turn right onto NY 23A and drive east about 11 miles. Just past Hunter, New York, bear right onto Bloomer Road, and then bear right again onto CR 16/Platte Clove Road. About 4 miles later, keep your eye out for Prediger Road, on the right. Turn right, and then follow the road right past a few private residences to a trailhead with ample parking (42° 8.0391' N, 74° 6.2541' W).

OVERNIGHT OPTIONS

Camping is tightly regulated along Devil's Path, and the relative scarcity of flat ground and water means that you'll have to sequence your campsites carefully. Camping is prohibited above 3,500 feet or within 150 feet of shelters, streams, or trails. Given the ruggedness of the trail, you effectively only have a few places where you can camp.

Overlook Shelter (turn off trail at 1.58/2,202/42° 07.143' N, 74° 05.253' W). About 1.58 miles in from the Prediger Road trailhead, Devil's Path swings right and climbs Indian Head Mountain. Walking south along Overlook Trail for a few yards, you'll soon come upon a lean-to near a creek. If you are arriving at the trailhead late, this shelter is an attractive option for getting an early jump on the trail the following day.

Mink Hollow Shelter (7.55/2,604/42° 08.129' N, 74° 09.753' W). In the notch after the precipitous descent from Sugarloaf Mountain, Devil's Path intersects with Mink Hollow Trail. Turn left (or south) for a lean-to. The sign indicates that there is a spring down Mink Hollow Trail to the north, but my party couldn't find it. Fortunately, you can find water a few hundred yards farther along Devil's Path, where a small stream crosses the trail.

Devil's Tombstone Campground (11.7/1,974/42° 09.206' N, 74° 12.469' W. Because it's situated close to the route's halfway point, where Devil's Path crosses NY 214, make use of the water pump as you cross the road. Then walk a few yards south along NY 214 to reach this campground, which offers an excellent overnight option for those walking the trail in two days. Be sure to book in advance. You cannot check in after 9 P.M., and the campground staff take this very seriously. Sites are $16 per night. 845-688-7160.

Devil's Acre Lean-to (13.8/3,508/42° 09.927' N, 74° 13.858' W). From NY 214, enjoy a long and often steep climb onto the southern shoulder of Hunter Mountain. At the top of the climb, you'll find a lean-to positioned near a water source.

Diamond Notch Falls (15.9/2,332/42° 10.491' N, 74° 15.470' W). Where Devil's Path passes through Diamond Notch, it crosses a beautiful stream and waterfall—ideal for soaking tired, aching feet, or perhaps going for a quick dip. Look around for tent sites, or walk about 0.5 mile south on blue-blazed Diamond Notch Trail to find the lean-to.

HIKE DESCRIPTION

From the Prediger Road trailhead, walk in on the red-blazed trail. You'll soon come across an intersection (0.25/2,073). Blue-blazed Jimmy Dolan Notch Trail heads off to the right, bypassing the first peak on Devil's Path. Bear left and follow the red blazes as the trail traverses gently through the forest. It arrives at an intersection with blue-blazed Overlook Trail (1.58/2,202). Devil's Path takes a hairpin turn to right and begins a steep and unforgiving climb up to Indian Head, which, at 3,573 feet, is the first of the peaks along this route.

Before you begin this climb, be sure to have sufficient water, as your next likely source is Mink Hollow (7.5/2,605), and your next certain source is NY 214 (11.5/2,003). Follow the blue blazes south to Overlook Trail shelter and its water source.

As you reach the shoulder of Indian Head (2.82/3,362), the Devil will treat you to the first of many excellent vistas along this route. But don't grow complacent. There's still more climbing to do. The trail heads down to a notch and then climbs steeply (including the longest stretch of Class 3 terrain on the route) to the summit, where a lovely view opens out (3.52/3,573/42° 6.9813' N, 74° 6.814' W). From this peak, the path descends sharply about 450 feet to

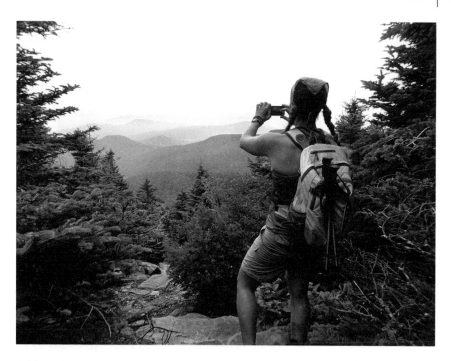

A hiker photographs a misty afternoon vista from Danny's Lookout along Devil's Path.

Jimmy Dolan Notch and the blue-blazed trail you passed by near the trailhead (3.94/3,114).

You'll quickly begin to understand how this trail earned its reputation. These descents are rugged and rocky enough that you will occasionally need to scoot on your posterior to down climb some of the more challenging rock chimneys and ledges. And then you will climb again, and then descend again. In this fashion, the summit of Twin Mountain (4.82/3,640/42° 7.5303' N, 74° 7.7515' W) gives way to Pecoy Notch (5.49/2,823). Then, Sugarloaf Mountain (6.41/3,800/42° 7.8832' N, 74° 9.02' W) drops off into Mink Hollow (7.5/2,605). This last descent of a mere 1,200 feet is particularly harrowing, as there are several sections of Class 3 terrain to clamber down. Take your time and be sure of each step. As you leave Mink Hollow, fill up your bottles before you climb to the summit of Plateau Mountain (8.52/3,840/42° 8.264' N, 74° 10.4987' W).

On the summit of Plateau Mountain, you may be forgiven for expelling a gasp of relief. The word "plateau" is not another demonic trick. Once the path crests this summit, you'll walk nearly 2 *flat* miles, passing the blue-blazed Warner Creek Trail on the left (8.9/3,783) and reaching spectacular views northward at Danny's Lookout and Orchard Point (10.4/3,673). At the latter, look left. Yes, that's the trail plunging off the plateau. After a descent of 1,700 feet—the longest on the trail—you'll reach NY 214 (11.5/2,003).

Cross the road, fill up your bottles at the pump, and then cross the little pond on the bridge. You'll soon be laboring your way up yet another climb. If it's any consolation, the west side of the path, while far from easy, is considerably less difficult than the east.

The trail takes a long climb up the southern flank of Hunter Mountain, alternating between rising steeply uphill and then switching back along a few ledges. Pass a stone outcropping that locals refer to as the Devil's Portal (12.2/2,757). Eventually, the trail levels out at about 3,500 feet and passes an intersection with yellow-blazed Hunter Mountain Trail (13.7/3,550). Devil's Path continues, passing by Devil's Acre Lean-to (13.8/3,508) and the side trail for the view at Geiger Point. Then, the trail begins its descent along West Kill Creek's drainage to Diamond Notch Falls (15.9/2,332).

Enjoy the alluring falls and the inviting swimming hole, especially during warm weather. Once you're done relaxing, however, Devil's Path takes you up yet another long, sustained climb—almost the last one. After climbing steeply, the path eases off along a ridgeline, but still ascends more gently to a series of impressive southward views (18/3,826) and then the true summit of West Kill Mountain, which, at 3,880 feet, is the highest point along the trail (18.2/42° 10.0967' N, 74° 17.3527' W). Over the next 1.6 miles, the trail descends fairly gradually, but treats you to one final climb St. Anne's Peak (20/3,415/42° 10.2523' N, 74° 19.2653' W). From this point, it descends steeply, but not precipitously, into Mink Hollow's drainage, where the trail turns north (20.9/2,438).

Though boggy at times, the smooth downward grade of the last 1.4 miles of Devil's Path will feel like a blissfully normal trail. At first, the trail follows the creek on its east bank, but then rides up onto the knees of the mountain before returning you to your vehicle on Spruceton Road (22.2/1,830).

OTHER OPTIONS

If you're eager to add more miles to this devil of a hike, Escarpment Trail forms a horseshoe with Devil's Path that is linked together by Long Path. The presence of this latter thoroughfare, presently stretching north from the George Washington Bridge to Albany, means you could walk as many miles as you like in this region.

If you'd like to cut Devil's Path down into more easily walked pieces, you could take advantage of NY 214 to divide the trail into sections of 11.5 miles and 10.7 miles. Although the trail structure of the area does resist loops (unless you're willing to do a lot of road walking), you could make use of trails like Mink Hollow, Diamond Notch, and Overlook to design variants.

Some ambitious hikers also strive to complete Devil's Path in a single day. Even the strongest hikers will find this a worthy challenge.

NEARBY

Several of the local towns, such as Hunter, Tannersville, and Phoenicia, boast restaurants and businesses that will appeal to hungry backpackers. Woodstock is an especially attractive town that draws tourists. Tubing the choppy waters of the Esopus is, in the warmer months, a wonderful way to recover from a strenuous backpacking trip.

ADDITIONAL INFORMATION

For more information, visit the New York Department of Environmental Conservation at dec.ny.gov/lands/5265.html. In case of an emergency on the trail, call 877-457-5680.

TRIP 21
THE FJORDS OF NEW YORK

Location: Dix Mountain Wilderness Area, Adirondack Forest Preserve, New York
Highlights: Four 46ers (Dial, Nippletop, Colvin, and Blake), Fish Hawk Cliffs and Indian Head, Beaver Meadow Falls, and infinite views
Distance: 20.1 miles round-trip
Total Elevation Gain/Loss: 7,731 feet of gain/7,731 feet of loss
Trip Length: 2–3 days
Difficulty: Challenging
Recommended Maps and Other Resources:
- *High Peaks Trails,* 14th ed. ED. Tony Goodwin and David Thomas-Train. Lake George, NY: Adirondack Mountain Club, 2012. The map included with this book is especially valuable.
- USGS Quads: Keene Valley and Dix Mountain.

As you peer down the nearly thousand-foot drop into Lower Ausable Lake from Indian Head or Fish Hawk Cliffs, you'd be forgiven a flight of fancy that you are on the Norwegian coast, so sheer are the mountains, so deep the lake. Not only will you bag several 46ers (Adirondack peaks above 4,000 feet) along this route, but you'll also enjoy scenery of unsurpassed variety. If this is your first trip to the Adirondacks, you're likely to come away so thoroughly infatuated with this beautiful and challenging wilderness that you'll soon be plotting your next visit.

HIKE OVERVIEW

Starting from the St. Huberts trailhead, you'll hike into the high peaks of the Adirondacks, following a ridgeline that will take you to Dial and Nippletop, two of the 46ers that motivate so many hikers and backpackers in the region. After base camping in Elk Pass, you'll hike out-and-back to bag two more 46ers—Colvin and Blake—before starting a descent that will take you past several of the best sights in the Adirondacks. Fish Hawk Cliffs, Indian Head, Lower Ausable Lake, and Beaver Meadow Falls will each give you more than ample opportunity to fill your camera with breathtaking shots.

Though this trip is far from easy, it avoids much of the extremely rugged and demanding terrain for which the Adirondacks are so justly famed. It is thus an excellent introduction to some of the best hiking on the East Coast.

Because part of this route passes through the Adirondack Mountain Reserve's private land, you should be aware that they have additional rules beyond those for the wilderness areas: no dogs, camping, campfires, or swimming on land belonging to the club.

HOW TO REACH THE TRAILHEAD

The St. Huberts trailhead is easily reached fom I-87 in upstate New York: take Exit 30 and head north on US 9. After about 2.2 miles, bear left onto NY 73 and drive about 5.3 miles. Pass Round Pond, Chapel Pond, and the various turnoffs for the Giant Mountain Wilderness on your right. Turn left into the St. Huberts trailhead parking lot and park there (44° 8.97864' N, 73° 46.05198' W).

OVERNIGHT OPTIONS

Backcountry camping in the Adirondacks is highly regulated, more so than you may be used to in the Mid-Atlantic. You need to know the rules and follow them, and you should not be surprised to be visited by a ranger. The summary below is a start, but the latest information can be found at dec.ny.gov/outdoor/9198.html.

In the Dix Mountain Wilderness Area, group size should be limited to eight. Camp only at a designated campsite, and never camp above 4,000 feet. Though you are not required to use a canister in this area, you are encouraged to do so anyway. Canisters are heavy and cumbersome, but they work better than a bear line. If you do not use a canister, make sure to hang a bear line.

Elk Pass (7.6/3,328/44° 05.772' N, 73° 49.527' W). A narrow and uneven designated campsite at the base of the path's precipitous slope and near the shore of a lovely pond. This campsite will only accommodate a few tents, but it is the best-positioned spot available.

Gill Brook (turn off route at 14.14/2,550/44° 06.728' N, 73° 48.955' W). Along the red-blazed trail to Mount Colvin, you'll spot a few designated campsites beside Gill Brook, about 0.1 to 0.3 mile northeast past the yellow-blazed trail to Fish Hawk Cliffs. Though these campsites are less ideally positioned, they may be the best options if the Elk Pass site is taken or if you have several tents to pitch.

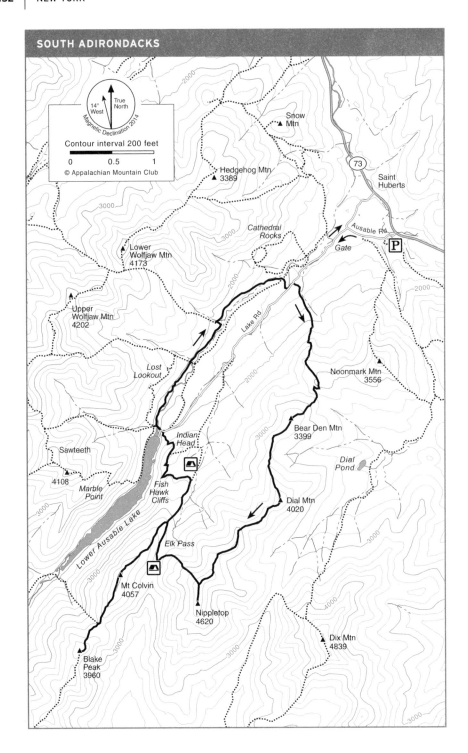

SOUTH ADIRONDACKS

14° West True North
Magnetic Declination 2014

Contour interval 200 feet

0   0.5   1
© Appalachian Mountain Club

Snow Mtn

73

Saint Huberts

Hedgehog Mtn 3389

Cathedral Rocks

Ausable Rd

Gate

P

Lower Wolfjaw Mtn 4173

Upper Wolfjaw Mtn 4202

Lake Rd

Noonmark Mtn 3556

Lost Lookout

Bear Den Mtn 3399

Dial Pond

Indian Head

Sawteeth

4108

Fish Hawk Cliffs

Dial Mtn 4020

Marble Point

Elk Pass

Lower Ausable Lake

Mt Colvin 4057

Nippletop 4620

Dix Mtn 4839

Blake Peak 3960

HIKE DESCRIPTION

As you leave the St. Huberts trailhead, the route passes through the private lands of the Adirondack Mountain Reserve until you're fairly far along the climb up Bear Den Mountain. Follow Ausable Club Road for almost 0.7 mile into the Ausable Club resort. Pass a sign, on the left, marking the trail to Noonmark Mountain (0.4/1,368) and walk by the golf course. Just as you reach the resort hotel, look for two tennis courts, and turn left onto Lake Road (0.66/1,361). Sign in at the trail register and walk through the gate (0.93/1,319).

About 0.7 mile farther along the road, a sign on the left of the trail marks the path to Bear Den Mountain, Dial, and Nippletop (1.62/1,446). This is Henry Goddard Leach Trail; follow it to begin the long, steady climb. Relish this trail, as it is much more gently graded than many in the Adirondacks. The route leaves the confines of the Adirondack Mountain Reserve, gains the shoulder of Noonmark Mountain, and treats you to a view of the Great Range from a ledge (3.0/3,021).

The trail then dips down to a notch where there is a water source (3.3/2,775) and climbs to reach the wooded and unremarkable summit of Bear Den Mountain (3.8/3,374/44° 7.1612' N, 73° 47.5985' W). Over the next 1.2 miles, the trail descends moderately to a col, and then climbs to the summit of Dial Mountain (4.9/4,020/44° 6.3453' N, 73° 47.7773' W), the 42nd highest peak in the Adirondacks. The next several miles undulate along this ridge-line, dropping down to cols before climbing to minor peaks. Eventually, the trail intersects with the blue-blazed trail that descends laboriously to Elk Pass (6.5/4,517). Before you take this trail, however, walk the 0.2-mile spur trail out and back to Nippletop (6.7/4,620/44° 5.3403' N, 73° 48.9838' W), which is the highest point of this trip. This view is reputed to be one of the best in the Adirondacks. Though Elk Lake is obscured from here, you'll be able to glimpse the Dix Range in the south and the Great Range to the north. Immediately ahead and below, you can see the ridgeline of Colvin and Blake.

Return to the intersection with the blue-blazed trail, and begin the tricky and often steep descent of 1,200 feet to Elk Pass. When I walked it, water trickled along the path, making it that much more imperative that each and every step be taken with care. This descent gives you a much stronger sense of the fabled difficulty of the Adirondacks. At the bottom, look for the designated campsite and the beautiful ponds in the pass (7.6/3,328).

Consider pitching camp here and walking out and back to bag Colvin and Blake. This trip is 5.3 miles, with about 2,440 feet of gain along rocky, challenging trails. You'll enjoy it most if you take plenty of time and go as light as possible.

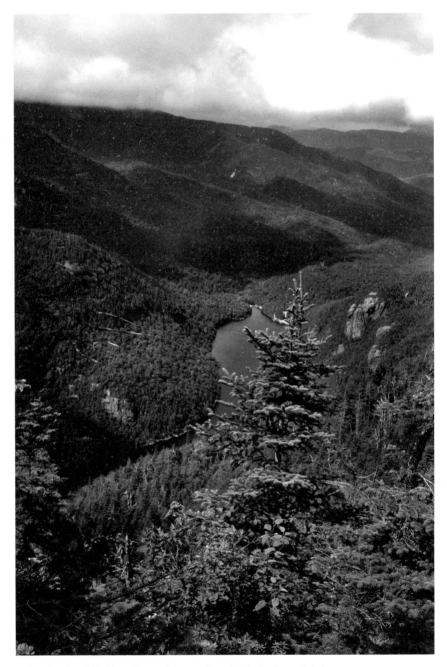

Enjoy the breathtaking views of Lower Ausable Lake from Colvin.

Leaving camp for Colvin, the trail passes between the two ponds and descends a few hundred feet to the junction with the red-blazed trail to Mount Colvin (8.2/3,236). You'll grieve for that lost elevation, as the climb up Colvin is the toughest bit of walking along this route. Turn left on the red-blazed trail and begin the often very rocky and steep climb to Colvin's summit. Just before reaching Colvin's summit, the trail turns left into a sheer wall that requires a tricky Class 3 move. Move right up to the wall and reach up to the right for a good handhold. Colvin's summit is just over this obstacle. Take in the jaw-dropping views of Lower Ausable Lake, far below, and the Great Range to the north (9.0/4,057/44° 5.6549' N, 73° 50.0735' W).

The next peak on your agenda is Blake, which is only 3,960 feet but—because of past surveying errors and love of tradition—is still considered one of the 46ers. After you've left the summit of Colvin, the trail proceeds along the fairly flat back of the ridgeline for a bit, but soon plunges steeply down to the col between Colvin and Blake (9.4/3,975). Two ladders aid your descent, but be careful, as they can be tricky to mount from above. From the col (9.7/3,436), the trail requires 0.5 mile and about 500 feet of climbing to reach the summit of Blake, which is unremarkable (10.2/3,960/44° 4.8769' N, 73° 50.6766' W). Another 0.5 mile farther along, Lookout Rock offers a better view for those who are not ready to retrace their steps.

Return to camp via Blake and Colvin, and enjoy a well-earned rest (13.0/3,328). The next morning, start the descent that features views that will rival even those from Colvin and Nippletop. Walk down, yet again, to the intersection with the trail to Colvin (13.6/3,236), but this time turn right and take the red-blazed trail down as it follows Gill Brook. It soon reaches a yellow-blazed trail on the left (14.1/2,550). Follow the yellow blazes to Fish Hawk Cliffs, where you'll have a wonderful view of Lower Lake Ausable from the sheer cliffs (14.6/2,462). As you leave this outcropping, climb rather steeply to reach a ridgeline. Turn left and walk out onto the cliffs of Indian Head, which tower 750 feet above the lake and offer a nearly panoramic view (14.8/2,653).

Following the yellow blazes, descend from Indian Head to Lower Lake Ausable. The trail soon arrives at Lake Road (15.5/2,026). Turn left for the dam at the foot of the lake. Once again, you're on private land, so there's no swimming in this very inviting lake. At this point, you have a few options for following the East Branch of the Ausable River down toward St. Hubert. For a charming and picturesque walk down the Ausable, cross the river here on the suspension bridge and take the yellow-blazed West River Trail.

As it heads northeast, the route immediately passes trails leading westward to Sawteeth and Pyramid (15.8/1,968). Continue to follow yellow blazes. The

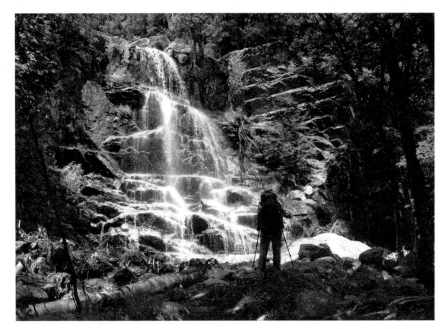

The cascades of Beaver Meadow Falls encourage a few moments of contemplation.

trail passes an open area known as Beaver Meadows, then arrives at Beaver Meadow Falls—as beautiful a waterfall as any in the region (16.7/1,939). Farther along, the trail crosses a bridge over Wedge Brook (an appealing cascade is up a side trail a short distance; 17.4/1,830) and shadows the Ausable River as it becomes even more gorge-like and full of raging whitewater. You might imagine yourself in the Himalayas.

Take the suspension bridge over this torrent (18.1/1,461) and follow the forest road downstream. It soon joins up with Lake Road (18.5/1,439). Pass the trail to Bear Den Mountain on the right and know that you've come full circle (18.6/1,422). Walk 1 mile out to the gate, turn right, and continue 0.7 mile to reach your vehicle (20.1/1,271).

OTHER OPTIONS

Given the impressive trail network in the High Peaks region, it's tempting to wander and explore so long as your food holds out. In fact, it's hard to walk along the Lower Ausable and ignore the many "quick" out-and-back possibilities to climb more peaks. Strong backpackers looking for an ambitious route might choose to carry their gear over Colvin and Blake, camp at the designated site beneath Pinnacle, and then swing around Elk Lake to the Dix range. With a potential total of nine 46ers along this extended route (some off-trail), this tempting trip should only be taken by expert backpackers.

NEARBY

If you're looking for fun and entertaining après-hike activities, you won't have to look far in the Adirondacks. Keene, Keene Valley, and Lake Placid are all located nearby, and they offer a full range of services for the backpacker in need of a little R&R from the trail.

ADDITIONAL INFORMATION

For additional information about the Adirondacks, visit the website of the New York Department of Environmental Conservation at dec.ny.gov/lands/9164.html and the website of the Adirondack Mountain Club at adk.org. Another great resource may be found at adkhighpeaks.com. In the event of an emergency, call the Department of Environmental Conservation's 24-hour hotline at 518-891-0235.

TRIP 22
ADIRONDACKS THE GREAT

Location: Eastern High Peaks, Adirondack Forest Preserve, New York
Highlights: Eight 46ers (including the Great Range and Mount Marcy), Lake Colden, Avalanche Lake, Heart Lake, and the Brothers
Distance: 39.7 miles round-trip
Total Elevation Gain/Loss: 12,512 feet of gain/12,512 feet of loss
Trip Length: 4–6 days
Difficulty: Epic
Recommended Maps and Other Resources:
- *High Peaks Trails,* 14th ed. ED. Tony Goodwin and David Thomas-Train. Lake George, NY: Adirondack Mountain Club, 2012.
- USGS Quads: Keene Valley and Dix Mountain.

Stupendous views from the Great Range, crystalline lakes carved deep into granite gorges, raging torrents, demanding scrambles, and precipitous descents: this trip has everything to tempt the expert backpacker. It also has the virtue of serving as a comprehensive circumnavigation of the high peaks of the Adirondacks. Walk this route and you'll likely return home dreaming of the mountains you didn't climb. You'll soon be scheming to return for more!

HIKE OVERVIEW

Standing atop Big Slide's summit ridge on a clear day, you'll be able to survey the grand loop you've walked around the eastern region of the Adirondack's high peaks. Across the valley of Johns Brook, you'll enjoy a capital view of the Great Range, including Lower and Upper Wolfjaw, Armstrong, Gothics, and Saddleback. In the distance, greater than the others, stands Mount Marcy. Away to the right, the bulk of Algonquin marks the valley you followed past Lake Colden and Avalanche Lake to reach Heart Lake, before climbing Klondike Brook to reach your current vantage point. Over the remaining 3.3 miles, you'll descend over the series of rock ledges known as the Brothers to complete this circumnavigation of one of the grandest and most demanding wildernesses in the east, or anywhere.

Note that while dogs are allowed, four-legged hikers aren't well suited to take on the challenging scrambles throughout this route.

HOW TO REACH THE TRAILHEAD

For this loop, park at the Garden trailhead just to the west of Keene Valley. From I-87 in upstate New York, take Exit 30 and turn left on US 9. In about 2.2 miles, bear left onto NY 73 and follow it for 8.3 miles into the town of Keene Valley. Turn left on Adirondack Road and follow the signs for the trailhead as the road takes you west into a residential area. The parking lot (which can become very crowded during peak times) is about 1.5 miles from downtown Keene Valley (44° 11.3405' N, 73° 48.9604' W). You'll be charged $7 per day to park a vehicle here.

OVERNIGHT OPTIONS

This entire route is in the Eastern Region of the High Peaks, so you'll need to be very conscious of the rules. Bear canisters are required April 1 through October 30. Limit groups to no more than eight. Camp in designated campsites only. No campfires. Obtain a self-issuing permit at the trailhead. Always follow Leave No Trace guidelines. And, finally, do not be surprised if a ranger visits your campsite to check compliance with these rules. Remember to check dec. ny.gov/outdoor/9198.html for the most up-to-date regulations.

Despite these restrictions, there are many very attractive options for camping and lodging while on this trip, including the very civilized option of staying at the Adirondack Mountain Club's lodges, which can give your trek almost the feel of hiking between European huts or mountain stations.

Ore Bed Shelter (10.6/2,767/44° 08.397' N, 73° 51.860' W). After Saddleback and Gothics, you may be eager for a rest. If so, consider spending the night at this lean-to along Ore Bed Trail. A designated campsite is available nearby, if you prefer your tent.

Johns Brook Lodge (12/2,324/44° 09.502' N, 73° 51.748' W). In this section of the Adirondacks, all trails do lead to the Johns Brook Lodge, so you're very likely to spend at least one night in its proximity. Take your pick between tent camping nearby, sleeping in the lodge, or renting a cabin. Visit adk.org to learn more.

Opalescent River (20.9/3,269/44° 06.878' N, 73° 57.336' W). From the four-way intersection with the trails to Skylight and Marcy, head westward, reaching a blue-blazed trail (heading northeast toward Colden) and a yellow-blazed trail to the southwest. Both trails have shelters and designated campsites nearby.

Lake Colden (22.7/2,771/44° 07.0771' N, 73° 59.0091' W). When you reach the lake, cross the outflow of the Opalescent River to find a number of campsites as well as a lean-to. You might be best served, however, by exploring

HIGH PEAKS

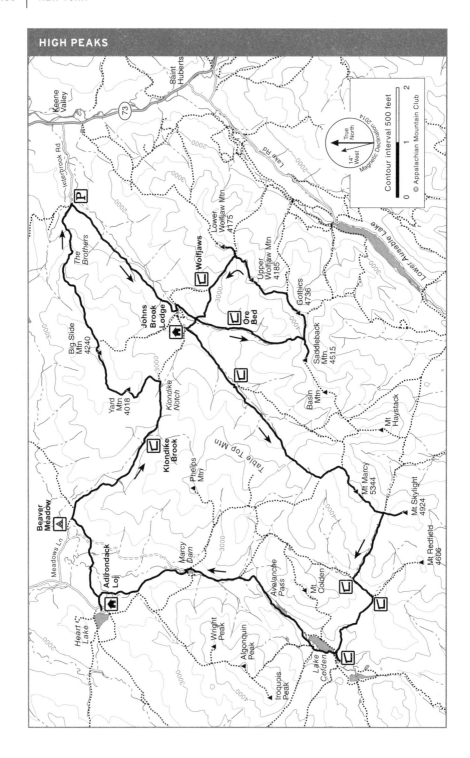

Keene Valley

Saint Huberts

73

Interbrook Rd

P

The Brothers

Lower Wolfjaw Mtn 4175

Lake Rd

Wolfjaws

Upper Wolfjaw Mtn 4185

Gothics 4736

Lower Ausable Lake

Johns Brook Lodge

Ore Bed

Saddleback Mtn. 4515

Big Slide Mtn 4240

Basin Mtn

Mt Haystack

Yard Mtn 4018

Klondike Notch

Klondike Brook

Phelps Mtn

Table Top Mtn

Mt Marcy 5344

Mt Skylight 4924

Beaver Meadow

Meadows Ln

Adirondack Loj

Marcy Dam

Avalanche Pass

Mt Colden

Mt Redfield 4606

Heart Lake

Wright Peak

Algonquin Peak

Lake Colden

Iroquois Peak

Contour interval 500 feet

True North

14° West

Magnetic Declination 2014

© Appalachian Mountain Club

0   1   2

some, as there are a number of beautiful campsites and lean-tos surrounding Lake Colden, a few with outstanding views.

Heart Lake (28.8/2,177/44° 10.968' N, 73° 57.842' W). No matter how you walk this loop, plan to spend a night near Heart Lake, which, apart from being a beautiful destination in its own right, offers you options for camping, including primitive sites and lean-tos around the lake, an established site suitable for vehicle camping, and, of course, the Adirondack Loj. More information is available at adk.org.

Klondike Brook (33.1/2,889/44° 10.0649' N, 73° 54.0481' W). A lean-to and a designated campsite are about 1.1 miles shy of the trail to Yard Mountain on your way up to Klondike Notch. This campsite gives you a good option if you want to spend one last night on the trail but are disinclined to descend to the Johns Brook Lodge.

HIKE DESCRIPTION

From the trail register and the Garden parking lot, begin following the yellow-blazed Phelps Trail toward the Johns Brook Lodge. The path is broad and well worn, and though it climbs slightly in sections, it is fairly flat. The trail passes a turnoff for Southside Trail, which provided an alternate route to the lodge but has been closed due to storm damage (0.5/1,660). Cross several brooks and pass by two shelters and a few campsites before arriving at the New York State Department of Environmental Conservation (DEC) Interior Outpost (3/2,210). Bear left to cross a suspension bridge over Johns Brook. It may be worthwhile to have your map in hand, as there are quite a few trail intersections in the vicinity of the lodge.

On the south side of the brook (3.1/2,211), turn right on the blue-blazed Ore Bed Trail and walk southwest about 0.4 mile before you reach an intersection (3.5/2,459). Note this intersection well, as you'll come to this point again after descending Ore Bed Trail from Saddleback and Gothics. For now, you'll turn left and begin climbing yellow-blazed Woodsfall Trail. When the trail reaches a rock slide to traverse, it's about to intersect ADK Range Trail (4.2/2,693). Campsites and a shelter are nearby, but more importantly, you should top off your bottles in the nearby Wolfjaw Brook. After you climb this valley, you won't encounter a certain source of water again until you descend from Saddleback—about 5 hard miles later.

Turn right and begin a steady climb up the ridge of the Great Range, with Wolfjaw Brook on your left. The brook peters out, and the trail arrives at the saddle between Lower Wolfjaw on the left and Upper Wolfjaw on the right (5.0/3,469). Here, you'll intersect with the yellow blazes of the trail that follows the Great Range, both to the northeast and the southwest. Start your exercise in peak-bagging by walking out-and-back to visit Lower Wolfjaw; you could drop your packs here for the 0.7-mile round trip, if you like. Along the way, the trail passes the blue-blazed Wedge Brook Trail leading down to the Ausable River on the right (5.1/3,615). Continue to follow the yellow blazes to the summit of Lower Wolfjaw. The distance to this summit is not far, but it offers a taste of the challenge the Great Range will offer, as there are a number of steep, Class 3 pitches. Lower Wolfjaw is the least remarkable summit you'll see on this route (5.4/4,175/44° 8.8898' N, 73° 49.9784' W), but if you peer out from its viewpoints, you'll spot Big Slide Mountain and the Brothers on the opposing ridge. You'll descend them at the end of the trip.

For now, descend back to the saddle (5.7/3,525), grab your pack, and start the climb to Upper Wolfjaw, following yellow blazes that ascend steeply up over a number of ledges—you'll certainly be using your hands to advance in many places. The trail passes a false summit (6.2/4,043), drops down to a col, and then ascends to a spur trail that leads to Upper Wolfjaw's summit—a broad ledge with a beautiful view to the south (6.5/4,185/44° 8.4246' N, 73° 50.7148' W). From here, you'll have an eagle's eye view at the highlights of Trip 21 in this book—Dial and Nippletop, Colvin and Blake, and Indian Head and Fish Hawk Cliffs, with Lower Ausable Lake below.

But the Great Range beckons, and the views will become ever more spectacular. Endure a quick but steep descent down into the col between Upper Wolfjaw and Armstrong (6.6/3,916). The climb of your next 46er begins with a ladder that takes you over a nearly vertical rock face, but the trail won't let up on you until you're standing on the summit rock of Armstrong (7.1/4,400/ 44° 8.0706' N, 73° 50.9822' W), where you'll enjoy an awe-inspiring view of the upper Great Range ahead of you: Gothics, Saddleback, Basin, Haystack, and above them all, Marcy.

The trail drops down to the col between Armstrong and Gothics and passes a blue-blazed trail that heads south to the dam on Lower Lake Ausable (7.4/4,409). Again, your yellow-blazed trail climbs steeply to reach the arctic-alpine zone, where the plants are especially fragile. Be sure to tread carefully and only on the rock. The amazing view from Gothics takes in dozens of major peaks (7.9/4,736/44° 7.6688' N, 73° 51.4387' W). When you're ready to move on, the path follows some flat walking along the summit, passes a blue-blazed trail to Pyramid and Sawteeth (8.07/4,650), and begins a very steep descent down the slabby west face of Gothics. Take your time, and use the cables. On grades like these, you'll be glad that Adirondack rock is so very grippy.

From the col between Gothics and Saddleback (8.5/4,053), drop your pack once again for the out-and-back to Saddleback's summit, now on blue blazes. The climb is steep but familiar by this point. Saddleback's summit is an excellent spot to take a break and enjoy what you've accomplished (9.1/4,515/44° 7.5805' N, 73° 52.4924' W). As you return to the col, be sure to look back at the face of Gothics and the steep slabs you descended.

Whether you intend to spend the night on the Ore Bed Trail, near the Johns Brook Lodge, or at Bushnell Falls, you have about 2,100 feet of descent ahead along Ore Bed Brook. Much work has been done on this section of trail, which was damaged by a number of rockslides caused by Hurricane Irene. The new path climbs down ladders, walks along steep slabs, and climbs down many newly constructed sets of stairs. At times, you may wonder if you're on the trail or in the brook. The Ore Bed shelter is on the right (10.6/2,767). From here, the grade is easier until you reach the Johns Brook Lodge area. Bear left on the yellow-blazed trail (11.7/2,392), cross the brook, and turn left at the lodge (12/2,324).

Your approach to Marcy will be a long one, as you follow yellow blazes southwest, keeping Johns Brook on your left. Eventually, the path intersects two trails that lead to Marcy (13.6/2,736). The red-blazed trail on the left climbs the peak by way of Point Balk and the col with Haystack; take the yellow-blazed trail on the right, which climbs Marcy after joining with the standard route coming in from Heart Lake and the Adirondack Loj. Before starting the long climb up through the forest, consider visiting Bushnell Falls via a steep trail down to the river.

After 2.7 miles and 1,800 feet of climbing, the yellow blazes bring you to blue-blazed Van Hoevenberg Trail (16.2/4,432), which runs north–south between Mount Marcy and the Loj. Turn left and begin the climb up Marcy. From this point forward, you'll have plenty of company as Van Hoevenberg Trail is well traveled. The trail soon turns slabby, and enters the arctic-alpine zone as the terrain opens out around you. The path climbs a small minor peak before finishing off the last ledges and slabs on the broad summit of Marcy (17.3/5,344/44° 6.7681' N, 73° 55.4141' W).

If the view from this great peak does not ignite your passion for climbing 46ers, then nothing will. Enjoy the 360-degree panorama and the broad sweep of wilderness, and note especially the line of the Great Range, much of which you climbed earlier in the trip. Pay particular attention to the broad peak to the southwest. This is Skylight, which is your next destination.

The descent from Marcy is slabby, but not nearly as steep as Gothics. Follow the blazes and stay off the vegetation; the path soon heads down over

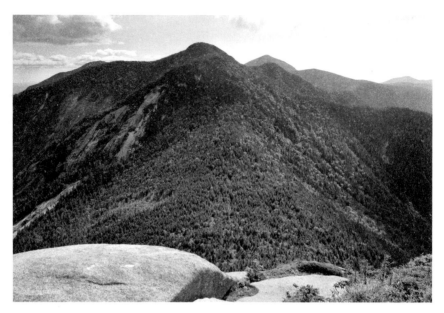

From Saddleback, backpackers will take in views of Basin and the upper Great Range.

Schofield Cobble and to the boggy area around Four Corners (18.1/4,361). To the left, a trail leads down to Panther Gorge; to the right, the yellow blazes take you to Lake Colden. First, continue straight ahead for a short climb to Skylight and yet another excellent view, including a great vantage of Marcy. This climb is steep and sometimes rocky (aren't they all?) until the trail opens out above tree line. Skylight's bare summit features more unobstructed views of the surrounding ranges (18.7/4,905/44° 5.9673' N, 73° 55.8695' W).

Return to Four Corners, then turn left and begin the 3.4-mile, yellow-blazed descent to Lake Colden. Pass Lake Tear of the Clouds on your right (19.3/4,328), then descend on a rugged, muddy, and rocky trail past an intersection with a blue-blazed trail on the right (20.3/3,362). This trail heads to Mount Colden and the Feldspar Lean-to, but you should continue to follow yellow blazes. At an intersection with a shelter and a number of trails (leading to Cliff and Redfield; 20.9/3,269), the blazes change to red and your route crosses a bridge.

Over the next 1.3 miles, the trail takes you along the southern bank of the Opalescent River. The footing may be rather messy and muddy in places, but the views of the raging river gorge are a real treat. Cross the Opalescent on a suspension bridge and reach Lake Colden (22.8/2,776); you'll almost certainly set up camp nearby.

The next section of trail is comparatively easy, and the scenery is a rare highlight in the Mid-Atlantic: beautiful lakeside walks around Lake Colden and Avalanche Lake. Cross Lake Colden on the suspension bridge and walk past the many campsites and the DEC Interior Outpost as the trail rounds the west shore of the lake. Pass intersections with yellow-blazed trails, one leading to Cold Brook Pass and Indian Pass (23.2/2,775), the other to Algonquin (23.3/2,774). Eventually, take a yellow-blazed trail that climbs northeast from Lake Colden to Avalanche Lake.

The next 2 miles of trail are some of the most beautiful in the Adirondacks, as your route crosses the foot of Avalanche Lake and makes its way along its westernmost shore. To the right, the sheer face of Mount Colden rises. The western shore is no less sheer, and the trail makes its way by scrambling over boulders, scampering down ladders and, at two points, running along catwalks bolted into the rock walls; this is beautiful and rugged terrain indeed (24/2,866).

Once you've passed the "Hitch Up Matilda"—so named for a woman who had to be carried over this path and was immortalized by a drawing in *Harpers*—the trail is easier to Heart Lake and the Adirondacks Loj. Descend along Marcy Brook, cross the stream beneath the remnants of Marcy Dam (26.6/2,361), and have increasingly gentle walking as you pass the standard route for Algonquin on the left and, at last, reach the information center at Heart Lake (28.8/2,177).

From the Adirondack Loj, proceed south through the parking lot where day-hikers gear up for Marcy and continue a few yards south until you reach an intersection with Mr. Van Ski Trail (red blazed) on the right (29.1/2,179). Over the next 1.8 miles, walk this unmaintained ski trail to join up with Klondike Trail and begin your trek back to the trailhead. Unfortunately, this section of trail is haphazardly blazed, marshy, and just plain tough going. In particular, you'll cross Marcy Brook, which could spell trouble in times of high water (29.7/2,052). Once on the opposite bank, look to the right to pick up the trail. Cross the broad and well-trodden South Meadows truck trail (30.3/2,091), then press on to reach red-blazed Klondike Trail (30.9/2,107).

Turn right and begin climbing this trail as it ascends 1,120 feet over 2.9 miles through the forest, passing an attractive shelter and campsite (33.1/2,889). When the trail reaches Klondike Notch (33.7/3,137), it descends for a few minutes to the intersection with the blue-blazed trail leading to Yard Mountain (35.2/4,018). A rocky, steep climb follows to this unremarkable summit, which is high enough to be a 46er but too close to Big Slide. The blue blazes descend slightly to a col, but then take a gentle climb to the beautiful vantage point from Big Slide's summit (36.4/4,240/44° 10.9287' N, 73° 52.2517' W).

In addition to this wonderful view from your last 46er on this route, your descent to your vehicle will feature a number of superb views from the rocky ledges known as the Brothers. The trail descends steeply from the top of Big Slide, passes a red-blazed trail leading back to the Johns Brook Lodge (36.6/3,833), and then descends more moderately as you pass the three Brothers, one after the other, each offering varied and stunning views of the valley and the range (38/3,128). After you've negotiated these final ledges and slabs (38.8/2,396), the trail dips down into the forest and the blue blazes will take you to your waiting vehicle (39.7/1,523).

OTHER OPTIONS

As ambitious as this backpacking trip is, the high peaks afford you ample scope for making it even more epic. If you spend much time in the Adirondacks, you'll hear hikers talking about a Great Traverse, hiking the series of peaks beginning with Rooster Comb, then summiting in turn Hedgehog, Lower Wolfjaw, Upper Wolfjaw, Armstrong, Gothics, Saddleback, Basin, Haystack, and Marcy. Including a Great Traverse on this route would have an advantage: it would save you from losing all the elevation along Ore Bed Trail that you must regain climbing back to Marcy. You might camp at Sno-Bird, a high campsite on the backside of Basin.

But be warned. Such a route should only be undertaken by the most experienced and fittest of backpackers. One particular challenge is a climb down a series of ledges on Saddleback's west side that offers several hundred feet of exposed Class 3 terrain. You should be a confident scrambler with minimal weight on your back.

Similarly, instead of walking through Avalanche Pass, you might opt to climb Algonquin and bag Iroquois, Boundary, and Wright before descending to Adirondack Loj at Heart Lake. You'll be trading the beautiful lakeside walk for more peaks, but there's enough terrific scenery on this route to motivate more than one visit.

NEARBY

With all the great restaurants and shops of Keene, Keene Valley, and Lake Placid nearby, you're not going to hurt for ways to occupy your time before, after, or between backpacking trips.

ADDITIONAL INFORMATION

New York's Department of Environmental Conservation (dec.ny.gov/lands/9164.html), the Adirondack Mountain Club (adk.org), and the forums at adkhighpeaks.com are all essential resources for exploring this magnificent wilderness. If an emergency occurs, contact the Department of Environmental Conservation at 518-891-0235, even before calling 911.

TRIP 23
GIANT STEPS

Location: Giant Mountain Wilderness, Adirondack Forest Preserve, New York

Highlights: Amazing views of the Lake Champlain Valley, Mary Louise Pond, and Rocky Ridge Peak and Giant Mountain

Distance: 9.9 miles one-way

Total Elevation Gain/Loss: 5,555 feet of gain/4,549 feet of loss

Trip Length: 2–3 days

Difficulty: Strenuous

Recommended Maps and Other Resources:
- *High Peaks Trails,* 14th ed. ED. Tony Goodwin and David Thomas-Train. Lake George, NY: Adirondack Mountain Club, 2012.
- USGS Quad: Elizabethtown.

Often vaunted as one of the best walks in the Adirondacks, this tough but rewarding ridge walk passes through open high country where the 360-degree views follow one after another in a way that quickly spoils Mid-Atlantic hikers. Walked in autumn, when the mountains a riot of fall color, this hike could compete with the best of the best. Of particular note are the views from Giant Mountain and Rocky Ridge Peak.

HIKE OVERVIEW

From NY 9 to NY 73, this route takes you westward on a traverse of the Giant Wilderness. You'll pass over Blueberry Cobbles and Bald Peak before camping high (just under 4,000) at Mary Louise Pond—a rare treat in the Adirondacks. Few views could be more beautiful than sunset from above this pond. On the next day, you'll bag Rocky Ridge Peak (4,420) and Giant Mountain (4,627) before completing the beautiful but challenging descent—3,100 feet in 2.6 miles. Giant steps, indeed.

HOW TO REACH THE TRAILHEAD

This route requires a vehicle shuttle, but the distance between the starting point and ending point is relatively short. From I-87 in upstate New York, take Exit 30 and head north on US 9. After about 2.2 miles, bear left onto NY 73 and drive about 3.8 miles. Just before you pass Chapel Pond, look for the trailhead marked for Giant Mountain and pull off on bays alongside the road (44° 8.285' N, 73° 44.617' W).

Leave one vehicle here, then return southward on NY 73 to the intersection with US 9. Bear left onto US 9, and drive about 4.5 miles north along the Bouquet River. You'll spot a trailhead parking lot for the Giant Wilderness on the left (44° 8.9866' N, 73° 37.6052' W). Pull in, park, and sign the trail register.

OVERNIGHT OPTIONS

The Giant Mountain Wilderness Area is distinct from the more restrictive Eastern High Peaks Zone, so the rules are a little different. Using bear canisters is not required, but it is encouraged. You should limit group sizes to eight and camp only in designated areas. Campfires are allowed, but do take care.

Mary Louise Pond (5.4/3,924/44° 09.323' N, 73° 41.783' W). At just under 4,000 feet, this designated campsite is one of the highest and one of the best in the High Peaks Region. Camping here may be one of the most persuasive arguments for backpacking this route, as the pond itself is quite beautiful and you will have easy access to stunning views, especially at dawn and dusk. Look for spur trail access on the left from your yellow-blazed route as you draw near the pond. The campsite has room for a number of tents.

Giant Washbowl (9.2/2,293/44° 08.513' N, 73° 44.322' W). If you choose to do two nights on this trail, use this beautiful designated site near NY 73. You reach the lake after your descent from Giant; designated campsites are to the left. Camping is not allowed on the shores of the lake.

HIKE DESCRIPTION

The sign at the trailhead reminds hikers of the 8 miles and 5,300 feet required to summit Giant Mountain. While the distance is not long, the verticality of the terrain tests even very strong backpackers. Make sure you're carrying enough water to reach Mary Louise Pond in 5.4 miles, as that is your only certain water source until you approach NY 73 on the far western side of the traverse.

From the trailhead, the yellow-blazed East Trail takes you through a forest of evergreens at a fairly moderate grade, but it soon becomes much more serious about climbing to Blueberry Cobbles. Many views of the Bouquet River valley open up behind you (1.55/1,743). A little farther along, a red-blazed trail allows you to detour around the cobbles, but you should follow the yellow blazes up and over this prominence (2.07/2,054). In late summer, you can devour the blueberries that line the trail while your eyes feast on views that grow more dramatic with every footstep. The trail drops down quickly to Mason Notch, where the red-blazed trail ends its detour (2.25/1,904).

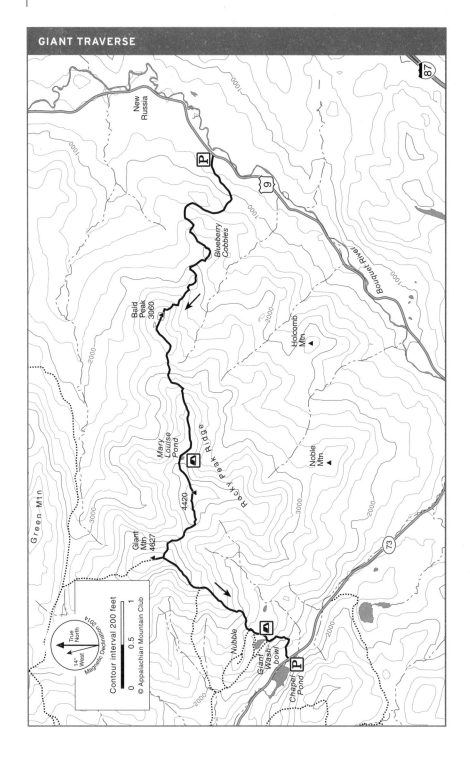

GIANT TRAVERSE

Over the next 1.24 miles, the yellow-blazed trail takes you to the summit of Bald Peak, climbing first to the summit of a minor peak, dropping down slightly, and then beginning a steep, slabby climb to the top of the mountain (3.5/3,027/44° 9.5558' N, 73° 39.8608' W). You'll be rewarded with a 360-degree panorama of the area. To the east, the thin, blue line of Lake Champlain is visible, and beyond it, Vermont; to the west, you can glimpse your route as it climbs Rocky Peak Ridge and then veers slightly north to reach Giant.

From the summit, the trail drops 500 feet into a forested area (4/2,752) before beginning a 1,200-foot climb to the eastern end of the ridge of Rocky Peak. It crosses several ledges before reaching the bare summit (4.9/3,988/44° 15.4175' N, 73° 42.3029' W). As you make your way along this ridge, enjoy open views before you arrive at Mary Louise Pond, where the designated campsite is located off a spur trail on the left (5.4/3,921).

The yellow blazes take you around the pond to the right and climb toward the summit of Rocky Ridge Peak. Be sure to look back toward the pond, as the views from above are truly impressive. Once you reach the summit, you'll be standing atop the twentieth-highest peak in the region (6/4,420/44° 9.245' N, 73° 42.303' W). Views are available in all directions. To your northwest, Giant Mountain looms.

The yellow blazes descend quickly to a notch between the two 46ers (6.63/3,743), and then start the last steep climb to the summit of Giant—900 feet over 0.6 mile—featuring some relatively vertical scrambling moves. When you encounter the blue-blazed trail coming in from the left (7.08/4,530), make a mental note—this is your route down. In just a few minutes more, you summit Giant (7.2/4,627/44° 9.6644' N, 73° 43.2092' W), with stupendous westward views of Dix and the Great Range. At 4,627 feet, Giant is the twelfth-highest peak among the 46ers. Time to soak it in.

From the summit of Giant, return to the blue-blazed trail and descend to NY 73. The descent isn't especially long (about 2.6 miles), nor is it the toughest in the Adirondacks. It is, however, quite sustained, losing about 3,100 feet in that distance. The grade is moderately steep for the first 0.6 mile to the intersection with Roaring Brook Trail on the right (7.8/4,045). Continue to follow the blue blazes down, on the left, now Zander Scott Trail.

As the descent continues, you'll arrive at slabs permitting excellent views of Giant Washbowl and Chapel Pond, below and to the west (8.64/3,077). A more modern trail switchbacks down to the lake and its designated campsites (9.2/2,293); pass them on the left, then reach an overlook of the valley below (9.3/2,295). The trail continues to descend, sometimes steeply, through a

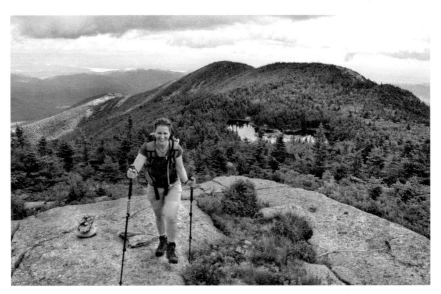

A hiker climbs for Rocky Ridge Peak after leaving camp at Mary Louise Pond.

forested area. Cross a small brook and reach NY 73 and your waiting vehicle (9.9/1,614).

OTHER OPTIONS

Whether you do this trip over one or two nights, it could make sense to reverse it, hiking west from NY 73 to NY 9. Also consider using the Roaring Brook trailhead, which will take you past a striking waterfall. A number of designated campsites in the vicinity of NY 73 make walking in late on Friday night an option.

NEARBY

The local towns of Lake Placid, Keene, Keene Valley, and Saranac Lake will not disappoint backpackers looking for a pint, a quick bite to eat, or a replacement for a forgotten or broken piece of equipment.

ADDITIONAL INFORMATION

A number of great resources provide ample information about the Adirondacks, including the website of the New York Department of Environmental Conservation at dec.ny.gov/lands/9164.html, the website of the Adirondacks Mountain Club at adk.org, and the forums at adkhighpeaks.com. In the event of an emergency, call the Department of Environmental Conservation's 24-hour hotline at 518-891-0235.

5

MARYLAND

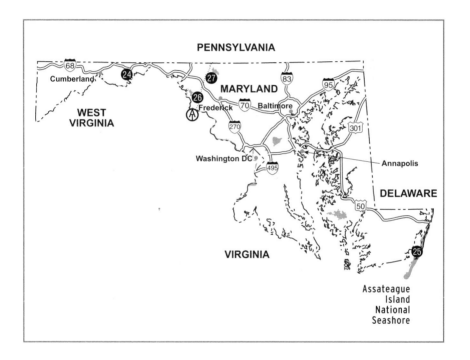

PENNSYLVANIA

68 Cumberland 24 27 MARYLAND 83 95

26 Frederick 70 Baltimore

WEST VIRGINIA 270 301

Washington DC 495 Annapolis

DELAWARE

50

VIRGINIA 25

Assateague
Island
National
Seashore

TRIP 24
ACROSS THE RIVER, THROUGH THE WOODS, AND *UNDER* THE MOUNTAIN

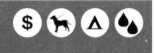

Location: Green Ridge State Forest, Maryland
Highlights: Paw Paw Tunnel, C&O Canal, and Fifteenmile Creek
Distance: 42.3 miles round-trip
Total Elevation Gain/Loss: 4,491 feet gain/4,491 feet loss
Trip Length: 3–5 days
Difficulty: Moderate
Recommended Maps and Other Resources:
- *Green Ridge State Forest*, Maryland Department of Natural Resources, 2008.
- USGS Quads: Paw Paw, Oldtown, Artemas, and Flintstone.

Few trails in the Mid-Atlantic can boast of such varied scenery as this route through Green Ridge State Forest. The creek walks along Big Run and Deep Run; sections along the Chesapeake and Ohio Canal and the Potomac River; a passage though the Paw Paw Tunnel; and the pool and rock garden of Fifteenmile Creek will each surprise you and surpass your expectations. And while sections of this route are popular with hikers and cyclists, you'll experience marvelous seclusion by backpacking the entire loop. This gem in western Maryland may very well be the best kept backpacking secret in the state.

HIKE OVERVIEW

Starting at the visitors' center near I-68, this route takes you south along the Deep Run/Big Run and Log Roll trails to the Potomac River and the West Virginia border. You'll then walk 17 miles along the Chesapeake and Ohio (C&O) Canal as it follows the bends of the Potomac and complete the loop on Long Pond Trail. Both the most difficult and the most scenic trail in the Green Ridge, this last trail will take you along the beautiful south bank of Fifteenmile Creek.

Though a few sections of this route are challenging, they are counterbalanced by very easy walking along the canal. As a result, this is an excellent trip for intermediate backpackers looking to sample a rich variety of Mid-Atlantic delights.

HOW TO REACH THE TRAILHEAD

From the east, take I-70 west from Hagerstown, Maryland. About 25 miles later, take Exit 1A to merge onto I-68. After driving about 17 miles west on I-68, take Exit 64 for M.V. Smith Road. Take a right, and then another right onto Headquarters Drive. Park at the visitors' center (39° 39.9145' N, 78° 26.5348' W).

OVERNIGHT OPTIONS

You'll have a variety of places to camp along this route, including primitive sites, Adirondack shelters, and established campsites along the C&O Canal. Backcountry camping is permitted throughout the Green Ridge State Forest with a permit ($10 for up to six people, $1 for each additional person).

Adirondack Shelters The forest maintains shelters on Big Run/Deep Run Trail, north of Mertens Avenue (6.24/1,073/39° 36.415' N, 78° 29.321' W), just north of the C&O Canal on Log Roll Trail (13.0/751/39° 32.344' N, 78° 31.788' W), and where Long Pond Trail meets 15 Mile Creek (36.5/568/39° 39.134' N, 78° 24.592' W). Each of these sites has plenty of water, but the tenting sites nearby are limited. The Long Pond Shelter is quite popular.

Established Campsites along C&O Canal This route passes by a grand total of five established campsites along the canal: Purslane Run (19/517/ 39° 32.106' N, 78° 27.873' W), Paw Paw Tunnel (19.8/528/39° 32.687' N, 78° 27.663' W), Sorel Ridge (22.4/488/39° 34.542' N, 78° 27.470' W), Stick-pile Hill (26.9/472/39° 35.048' N, 78° 23.870' W), and Devil's Alley (31.6/449/ 39° 37.363' N, 78° 24.804' W). These sites are used by cyclists and boaters, and they are first-come, first-served. The Paw Paw Tunnel campground is the largest and most developed of these sites, while Purslane and Devil's Alley have more of a backcountry feel and enjoy views of the river. Each of these camp-sites has a pump with potable water. Contact the National Park Service for the most up-to-date information regarding fees at these sites.

Backcountry sites along Fifteenmile Creek You won't find as many primitive backcountry sites along the trails of Green Ridge as you might expect, though there's flat ground and often plenty of water. The best sites are found along the last few miles of Long Pond Trail (39.5/653/39° 39.760' N, 78° 26.624' W and 40.5/676/39° 39.494' N, 78° 26.779' W). Note that you could reach these sites at the beginning of the trip as well as the end. Much depends on how you want to sequence your campsites.

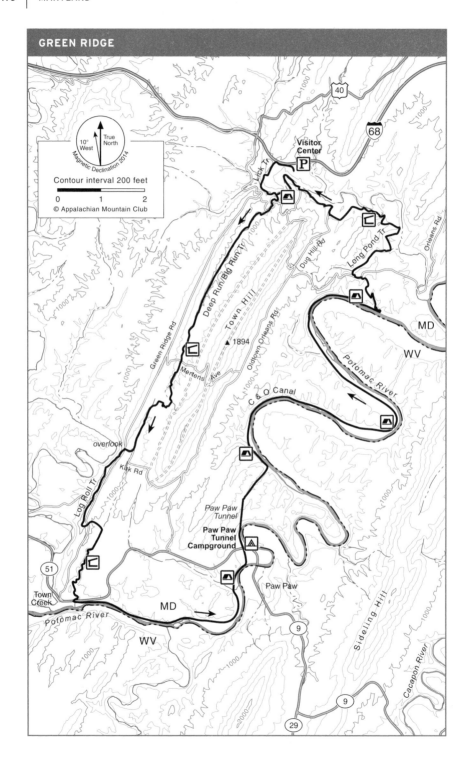

GREEN RIDGE

10°
West
True
North
Magnetic Declination 2014

Contour interval 200 feet

0   1   2
© Appalachian Mountain Club

Visitor
Center
P

40

68

Lick Tr

Long Pond Tr

Orleans Rd

Deep Run/Big Run Tr

Town Hill

Dug Hill Rd

MD

WV

Green Ridge Rd

Mertens Ave

Oldtown Orleans Rd

▲ 1894

Potomac River

C & O Canal

overlook

Kirk Rd

Log Roll Tr

Paw Paw
Tunnel

Paw Paw
Tunnel
Campground

Paw Paw

51

Town
Creek

Potomac River

MD

WV

9

Sideling Hill

Cacapon River

9

29

HIKE DESCRIPTION

Standing in the parking lot, look toward the restrooms. Just to the left is the placard marking the beginning of the route. Although the map marks this orange-blazed trail as Pine Lick Trail, it is really a spur trail leading about 1.2 miles to Pine Lick Trail. The spur takes you along some rolling terrain, sidles up to I-68 briefly, and then veers away to intersect with Pine Lick Trail (1.2/960). A right turn will take you to Pennsylvania; instead, turn left and begin a sharp and rocky descent down to an amusingly crooked footbridge over 15 Mile Creek (1.43/704).

Over the next half-mile, blue-blazed Pine Lick Trail rides up and down the western side of the creek's drainage. The path is occasionally fairly rugged, and there is even a spot with a scrambling move. Soon, though, it arrives at a fork (1.93/695). On the left, Long Pond Trail comes in from following Fifteenmile Creek—you'll be returning this way in a few days. For now, cross the creek on the fallen logs and take a right to head southward along the banks of Deep Run.

You'll soon come to a road (2.37/736); cross it, and look for the placard marking the beginning of Deep Run/Big Run Trail. You'll walk southward for the next 12 miles through the Deep Run Wildlands, a stretch of trail that is easy enough walking except for the countless crossings of Deep Run and later Big Run. By the time you reach the shelter just north of Mertens Avenue (6.24/1,073), you'll almost certainly have wet feet.

South of Mertens Avenue (6.5/1,099), you'll still have some crossings, but the walking will become very mild as the trail coincides more and more with an old road grade. At mile 9.3, you'll reach Kirk Road. Take a right and follow the road as it climbs up to Log Roll Overlook, with its beautiful view of Town Creek and pastoral western Maryland (9.54/1,117).

When you're ready to proceed, look for the orange blazes that mark Log Roll Trail a few feet south on Green Ridge Road. It dives off the ridgeline and then edges along the ridge for about 2 miles. Do keep your eye out for blazes along this section, as the trail occasionally turns away from the most obvious route. In good time, the path crosses Pack Horse Trail Road (10.9/1,102), turns eastward, and crosses Green Ridge Road (11.7/1,030). Log Roll Trail then descends to meet the southward-flowing Big Run (12.2/815). Many creek crossings ensue before you reach the shelter about 1.3 miles north of the Potomac (13/751).

The last few miles of walking along Big Run are some of the most rugged sections on the route, as the gorge becomes increasingly rocky and narrow and the trail takes perverse delight in crossing and recrossing the creek. A number

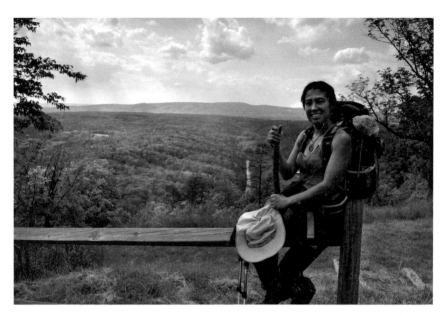

A hiker pauses to enjoy views of western Maryland from the Log Roll Trail.

of blowdowns may force you to bushwhack alongside the trail through a forest of bramble. With persistence, though, you'll soon emerge from this thicket on the banks of the Potomac.

Cross MD 51, and take a left (14.3/551). For the next 17 miles, walk along the C&O Canal's towpath, with the canal on your left and the Potomac on the right. Running 184.5 miles from Cumberland, Maryland, to Washington, D.C., the canal was constructed in the 1830s and 1840s as a means of bringing goods (especially coal from the Alleghenies) to the eastern seaboard. By the time the canal reached Cumberland in 1850, the railroad had beaten it by eight years, making it obsolete. Today, the park service maintains the canal for recreational purposes.

Because the canal is entirely flat and poses no navigational difficulties, walking along it is easy and pleasant. The miles—each marked by a post on the right—will fly by easily enough. But this stretch of hiking is far from monotonous. From the railroad trestles to the old stone locks, the transportation infrastructure of the nineteenth century offers plenty of picturesque scenes, and the canal itself is a haven for wildlife. Keep your eyes out for beavers, birds, snakes, frogs, and turtles that call the canal's still waters and banks home.

Pass Lock 67 and, as the canal bends north, arrive at the Purslane Run Campsite (19/517) and then the more developed Paw Paw Tunnel Campground (19.8/528), where MD 51 crosses the Potomac into West Virginia. Just ahead is the Paw Paw Tunnel (20.2/546), which cuts 3,118 feet into the mountain, allowing the canal to detour past six bends of the river. One of the great engineering feats of its day, it also nearly bankrupt the canal company. Break out your headlamp or flashlight and walk along the pathway, but be careful, as the pathway is uneven and wet in spots.

The canal emerges from the tunnel, passes several locks, and turns left once it regains the river (22/489). Follow the towpath as it continues to shadow the Potomac downstream, passing the Sorrel Ridge Campsites (22.4/488), the canoe campsites at Bonds Landing (26/483), and then finally, the Devil's Alley Campsite—a fine location for lunch or a nap (31.6/449).

Just past this campsite, the path reaches Lock 58. Look carefully for a placard indicating the junction with red-blazed Long Pond Trail (32/457), which you'll follow north. Cross over the little bridge on the lock and return to the forest on this trail, which starts you off properly with a steep little climb and switchbacks. Though this trail is the most challenging in Green Ridge, it is also some of the best walking.

Over a span of 4.2 miles, Long Pond Trail crosses the Potomac Bends Wildland to reach Fifteenmile Creek. First, it climbs about 500 feet to reach the Oldtown Orleans Road (33.4/930), where it takes a left. Walk until you see a placard on your right (33.5/856), then turn right. The trail descends quickly into the basin of Flat Run, which it follows for about 1.2 miles. Eventually, the trail turns left away from this creek (34.7/522), passes through some more open country, and begins to climb the ridgeline of the descriptively named "Big Ridge." This climb tops out (35.9/963) as Long Pond Trail starts a precipitous descent to Fifteenmile Creek (36.2/590); there are a few nice views along the way. The trail reaches the creek and turns west (left). Once at the creek, you'll quickly spot a few tent sites, the shelter itself (on a bluff to the left), and a number of very fine swimming holes. You'll want to explore here—Long Pond itself is downstream of where the trail meets the creek.

As Long Pond Trail proceeds westward, it climbs along some marshy old forest roads to meet Dug Hill Road (38/707). Though the map indicates that the trail cuts off a bend in the road, the blazes follow the road past a few primitive vehicle camping spots. Walk about 1 mile along the road, but keep your eye out for a right-hand turn away from the road and into the forest (38.9/701); it is easy to miss. Over the next few miles, Long Pine Trail drops down to meet Fifteenmile Creek, crosses tributaries, and then climbs back up above the creek. Each time the trail meets the creek, there are a number of very fine campsites. Your final dip will take you to the intersection with Deep Run and Pine Lick Trail, where your loop began (40.6/682).

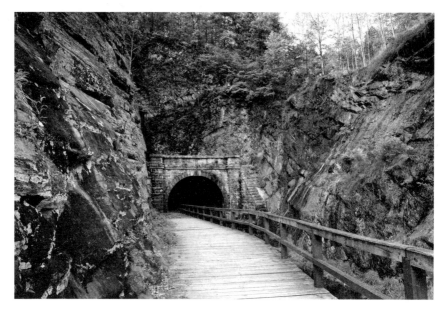

The Paw Paw cuts its way deep into the hills along the Potomac.

Use the log to cross Deep Run and head north on Pine Lick Trail, retracing your steps over the crooked bridge (41.1/710) and climbing to reach the intersection with the orange-blazed spur trail (41.4/963). Take a right here (if you cross I-68, you missed this turn) and return to the visitors' center and your vehicle (42.3/961).

OTHER OPTIONS

Although the forest managers are planning to add trails that would facilitate other circuits, at present you'll have difficulty walking a shorter loop without striking out along a road. Of course, an out-and-back trip is certainly doable. If you take advantage of the parking lot at the Paw Paw Tunnel Campground, you could divide this route into two sections for two weekends of backpacking.

If more miles are what you're after, then consider parking where Pine Lick Trail meets the Pennsylvania–Maryland border (also the beginning of Pennsylvania's Mid-State Trail) and hiking south to begin this route. Hiking a "tear-drop" loop of this sort will net you about 55 miles, and allow you to brag that you hiked across Maryland . . . twice.

NEARBY

Some of the little burgs (such as Paw Paw, West Virginia) along the C&O Canal provide services to the cyclists and hikers who enjoy the canal. The nearest large town is Hagerstown, Maryland, to the east, or Cumberland, Maryland, to the west.

ADDITIONAL INFORMATION

For additional information about Green Ridge State Forest, call 301-478-3124 or visit the forest's website at dnr.state.md.us/publiclands/western/greenridge forest.asp. You may purchase a map either online or at the visitors' center. To learn more about the C&O Canal, contact the National Park Service at 301-678-5463 or visit its website at nps.gov/choh/.

TRIP 25
DO YOU ENJOY LONG WALKS ON THE BEACH?

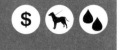

Location: Assateague Island National Seashore, Maryland and Virginia

Highlights: Backpacking along the beaches of a secluded and pristine Atlantic barrier island

Distance: 27.9 miles one-way

Total Elevation Gain/Loss: 320 feet gain/320 feet loss

Trip Length: 2–3 days

Difficulty: Moderate

Recommended Maps and Other Resources:

- National Park Service, Assateague Island National Seashore Maryland & Virginia, *Backcountry Camping Map*, 2008. nps.gov/asis/planyourvisit/upload/backcountrymap2008.pdf
- Potomac Appalachian Trail Club. "Assateague Island National Seashore." A valuable but out-of-date online resource, patc.us/hiking/destinations/assateag.html.
- *Abercrombie, Jay. Walks and Rambles on the Delmarva Peninsula: A Guide for Hikers and Naturalists (Walks & Rambles Guides).* Backcountry Publications, 1985.
- USGS Quads: Tingles Island, Whittington Point, and Chincoteague East.

With the waves crashing on the left and the sand dunes rising from the beach on the right, you're sure to feel the uniqueness of Assateague as soon as you start your walk along the Atlantic's ever-changing tideline. No matter how experienced an outdoorsperson you may be, you'll have a chance to see wildlife in this rich ecosystem that you may not have seen before—not just the famed wild horses, but 275 species of birds; a wealth of sea life such as horseshoe crabs, starfish, and sponges; and mammals like deer, red foxes, and river otters. This is one of those trips that every backpacker in the region needs to do at least once.

HIKE OVERVIEW

Backpacking a barrier island is an experience to relish, but it will test your skills in some interesting ways. More than other trips, enjoying your Assateague trip will hinge on how well you time your visit. If you go in the heat of summer, you may tell a tale of slogging through sand dunes in suffocating heat, battling clouds of mosquitoes, and enduring considerable off-road traffic on some portions of the beach. March or April is the ideal time to backpack Assateague.

Do not underestimate this trip; it's no easy walk on the beach! A well-worn adage states that "hiking 5 miles on Assateague is as strenuous as hiking 10–12 miles in the mountains," though I personally think it overstates the difficulty. Consider wearing trail runners, sport sandals, or even going barefoot some. Your feet will almost certainly get wet, and sand will get into your shoes. By the time you reach Tom's Cove, even the strongest backpackers will feel some unusual fatigue in their legs, and it's not uncommon to discover a strangely placed blister from walking on ground always sloped to the left

Consider carefully what you pack for this environment. There's no source of fresh water on the island, so bring all your water with you. The park service recommends about 1 gallon per person per day. In very hot weather, you're going to need more. Insects can also be a factor in backpacking comfort. Plan carefully to ensure 100 percent coverage, including carrying insect repellant, bringing a head net, and dousing your clothes in permethrin. Make sure your shelter is outfitted with netting. If you can, choose ocean-facing campsites, as the bay side is buggier.

Remember to wear sunscreen applied carefully and often. Walking next to the water increases your chances of sunburn, and backpackers tend to get burned in odd places once layers are removed or unzipped. Don't forget to apply thoroughly to the tops of your feet, too: a burn there could incapacitate you.

In addition to keeping up with weather alerts, check on the tides for your trip. A rising tide will usually make walking along the beach more difficult, while a retreating tide will make it easier. Check out tidesandcurrents.noaa.gov. This is essential information for a backpacking trip of this type.

From the moment you first set foot on this beach, with its miles and miles of undeveloped seashore, its pounding surf, and its wide expanse of sand dunes, you'll sense that this is a special place: this is one of the last barrier islands on the East Coast that is left, almost entirely, in its natural state. The route takes you from where the Verrazano Bridge ties Assateague to mainland Maryland to Tom's Cove in Virginia, covering 28 miles of some of the most secluded and pristine beach you'll ever encounter. Along the way, you'll enjoy wildlife

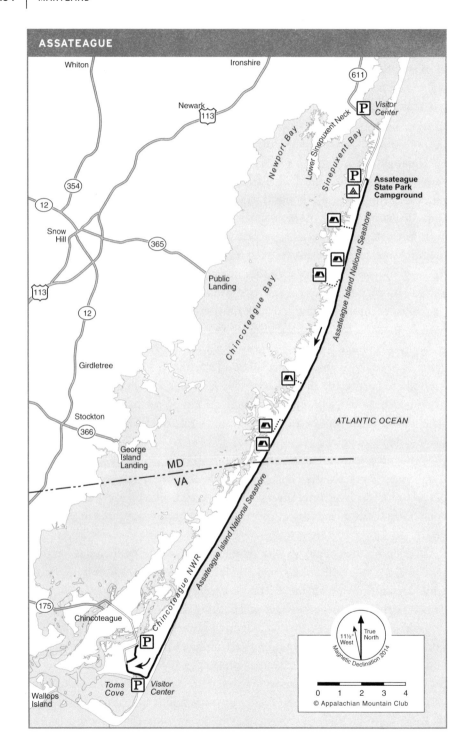

ASSATEAGUE

Whiton

Ironshire

611

Newark

113

Visitor Center

P

Newport Bay

Lower Sinepuxent Neck

Sinepuxent Bay

P

Assateague State Park Campground

354

12

Snow Hill

365

Public Landing

Chincoteague Bay

Assateague Island National Seashore

113

12

Girdletree

Stockton

366

George Island Landing

ATLANTIC OCEAN

MD

VA

Chincoteague NWR

Assateague Island National Seashore

175

Chincoteague

P

Toms Cove

P

Visitor Center

Wallops Island

True North

11½° West

Magnetic Declination 2014

0   1   2   3   4

© Appalachian Mountain Club

watching, superb opportunities for camping on the beach or on Chincoteague Bay, and incomparable beachcombing.

Access to Assateague can be more complicated than some national parks, but a careful plan for arrival, parking, and camping will keep your day-of worries to a minimum.

HOW TO REACH THE TRAILHEAD

To Reach the Ending Trailhead. From Salisbury, Maryland, drive south along US 13 for about 31 miles, passing the towns of Princess Anne and Pocomoke City, Maryland. After crossing the Virginia state line, take a left on VA 175 and proceed about 11 miles over the bridge spanning Chincoteague Bay. When you reach the town, continue straight on Maddox Boulevard. Go through a traffic circle (second exit), and then cross a bridge into the Chincoteague National Wildlife Refuge, where you'll enter the park via a gate (37° 54.660' N, 75° 20.965' W). Alert the person working the gate that you are planning to leave a vehicle for a backpacking trip and comply with the directions you're given. Go to the Tom's Cove Visitor Center, obtain a hanging permit, and park your vehicle in the location indicated by park staff. (Note that Tom's Cove Visitor Center is closed Tuesday through Thursday from December through February. If arriving when the center is closed, contact the ranger station for instructions.)

To Reach the Starting Trailhead. Head back out to VA 175 and turn north on US 13. Just before Pocomoke City, bear right on US 113. Continue north for 28 miles. Turn right on MD 376 just as you enter the town of Berlin. About 4 miles later, turn right onto MD 611. As you enter Assateague, get your backcountry permits at the ranger station on the island, next to the park entrance (38° 12.4478' N, 75° 9.1195' W). Comply with directions about where to park your vehicle.

To ensure that the Chincoteague National Wildlife Refuge gate is open (evening closing hours depend on the season) and that you have time to obtain any necessary camping permits (see below), time your arrival for morning or midday.

OVERNIGHT OPTIONS

The National Park Service maintains a number of attractive backcountry camping sites on the Maryland side of the seashore (camping is not allowed on the Virginia side of the state line). Because the rules surrounding the use of these campsites are quite complicated, you'll want to study the park service's website: nps.gov/asis/planyourvisit/backcountry-camping.htm. I also highly recommend that you contact the seashore prior to your visit, as you would not want to be surprised, on your arrival, by a sudden closure.

In brief, you'll need a backcountry permit to camp at any of these sites. The cost is low (just $6 per person), but permits are only issued on a first-come, first-served basis at the ranger station in Maryland or at the Tom's Cove Visitor Center in Virginia. Additionally, rangers will only issue you a permit if you are there in plenty of time to reach the campsite of your choice—you must request the permit the appropriate number of hours before sunset, based on your point of departure and your planned campsite:

For Maryland departures, apply for your permit for these campsites at least
- 2 hours before sunset for Tingles Island, Little Levels, and Pine Tree
- 4 hours before sunset for Green Run, State Line, and Pope Bay

For Virginia departures, apply for your permit for these campsites at least
- 4 hours before sunset for Pope Bay and State Line
- 6 hours before sunset for Green Run
- 8 hours before sunset for Pine Tree, Little Levels, and Tingles Island

Fines are in place for violating campsite restrictions. Illegal camping on the Maryland side of the line will cost you $175 per person, and $75 on the Virginia side. Contact the rangers and make sure you're complying with all rules.

The campsites offer two stunning choices of location—spending the night next to the bay or spending it next to the ocean.

Bayside Backcountry Sites: Tingles Island (2.3/38° 10.667' N, 75° 10.533' W); Pine Tree (spur trail at 4.75, campsite at 38° 8.600' N, 75° 11.300' W); Green Run (9.65/38° 4.800' N, 75° 12.812' W), and Pope Bay (12.0/38° 2.867' N, 75° 14.050' W). Walking along the ocean, you'll easily spot signs pointing you to these four idyllic sites. They are wooded and feature level ground perfect for tenting. Each site also features a fire ring, chemical toilet, a picnic table, and a great view of the sun setting over the bay.

Oceanside Backcountry Sites: Little Levels (4.0/38° 9.133' N, 75° 10.367' W) and State Line (12.5/38° 2.683' N, 75°13.883' W). These sites are perched in the dunes above the high tide mark. They too have picnic tables and chemical toilets, but ground fires are not allowed. Be wary of high tide, and come prepared to pitch your shelter in the sand (sand stakes may be in order).

Vehicle Camping at Assateague: If you're looking to rest after a long trek along the beach, you can enjoy the vehicle camping sites at the seashore. These sites include amenities like drinking water, cold showers, and chemical toilets. In the off-season, from October 16 through April 14, the sites are available first-come, first-served, and they cost $20 per night. In peak season, reservations are available and recommended. Higher fees apply. See recreation.gov.

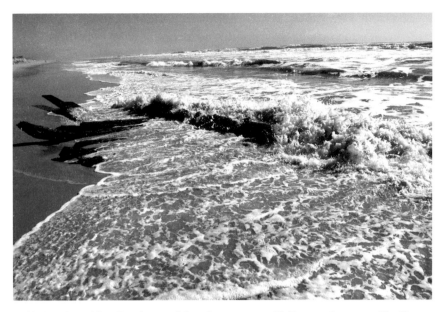

While beachcombing the shores of Assateague, you will discover treasures like these ancient timbers, washed up in the surf.

HIKE DESCRIPTION

From the parking lot, walk to the beach, turn right, and begin walking south along the tideline. The Maryland side of the path sports a long line of poles marching along the beach. Some of these poles are kilometer signposts, which correspond to the map the park service provides online.

Between the 17 and 18 kilometer markers, spot a trail leading to the Tingles Island bayside campsite (2.3). If you're walking in from the vehicles late in the afternoon, you may want to use this campsite, but in most cases, you'll want to walk on to Little Levels (4.0) or Pine Tree (spur trail at 4.75). By this point, you'll probably have caught sight of Assateague's most famed inhabitants, the wild horses that graze among its sand dunes. These animals are far from native to the island; in fact, they enjoy a legendary provenance. In the early nineteenth century, the merchantman *San Lorenzo* was returning to Spain from Peru when the ship was shattered off the coast of Assateague and driven onto the beach. Apart from the gold and silver of the Incas, in its hold were a number of ponies that had been bred to work in the mines and blinded to make them easier to handle. Somehow, a few of these hardy animals made it to shore and adapted to life on the barrier island. The wild horses you'll see along your journey are, it is thought, the descendants of these brave beasts. (Although these horses may, rather more prosaically, be the descendants of colonial animals pastured here to escape taxation in the 1600s, what is truly remarkable about them is their ability to thrive in the harsh conditions along the barrier island.)

Walk south past the spur trail for Green Run (9.65), then reach the spur trail for Pope Bay (12.2) and State Line campsite just beyond (12.5). Wherever you camp, be sure to ramble about after twilight; the wildlife of the island is rich, and you're more likely to catch a glimpse after the sun has set. There have even been reports of bioluminescent organisms in the surf.

Shortly after passing these campsites, you'll reach the fence (careful of its barbed wire, which can wreak havoc on delicate fabrics) marking the state line between Virginia and Maryland (14.4). Before you cross into Virginia, you'll see a few of the buildings that remain from when the Ocean Beach Corporation attempted to develop this pristine seashore into a housing tract with 5,850 lots, hotels, and shopping centers. Mother Nature was having none of it, and in 1962, a storm ravaged the island, ripping away roads and splintering houses. The government concluded that the cost of protecting the island from similar storms would be prohibitive, so the land was purchased for the park in the mid-1960s. If you ever happen to be out on Assateague during a particularly high tide, you'll have a glimmer of what such a catastrophic storm might look like. A few feet of surf would be more than enough to overtop the island.

Once you cross into Virginia, you'll be entering a paradise for beachcombers. There are no more campsites, no more kilometer posts, and no more vehicles, just 12 miles of splendidly isolated shoreline.

Hikers walking north from Tom's Cove are a sign that your trip is coming to an end. After reaching the visitors' center (25.5), take a left along the road, passing through the Chincoteague Wildlife Refuge as you return to your vehicle (27.9).

OTHER OPTIONS

Unlike a trip in the mountains, you can't add miles to this trip very easily, though it is sometimes possible to explore both north to the old washed-over campsite at Sinepuxtent or south around Tom's Cove. Check with the rangers, as these areas are closed, at times, due to overwash and nesting birds. A leisurely exploration of the dunes and bays of the islands will reward patience, and the beachcombing truly is excellent. If you're looking for a shorter trip, do an out-and-back trip from the Maryland side of Assateague. Given the proximity of the campsites at Tingles Island, Little Levels, and Pine Tree, you don't have to walk very far. A short trip of this type could easily appeal to a beginner backpacker.

If you'd like to rent a canoe, you can set out on an entirely different adventure by paddling along the bayside of the island.

NEARBY

Chincoteague has all the businesses you might expect of a coastal resort town. If you're looking for more amenities, Salisbury is the nearest large town along your route. It hosts several large outdoors stores if you've forgotten an essential piece of equipment. Ocean City and Berlin also offer equipment rentals.

ADDITIONAL INFORMATION

Contact Assateague Island National Seashore at 410-641-1441 for more information, or visit the website at nps.gov/asis/.

TRIP 26
VIEW FROM THE HEIGHTS

Location: Greenbrier and Gathland state parks, Maryland and Harpers Ferry, West Virginia
Highlights: Overlooks from White Rocks, Weverton Cliffs, and Maryland Heights; the dramatic entrance into Harpers Ferry; Civil War history
Distance: 24.7 miles one-way
Total Elevation Gain/Loss: 4,206 feet/5,142 feet
Trip Length: 2–3 days
Difficulty: Moderate
Recommended Maps and Other Resources:
- PATC, Maps 5 & 6, *Appalachian Trail across Maryland and the entire Catoctin Trail*. August 2009.
- *Appalachian Trail Guide to Maryland and Northern Virginia, With Side Trails*, 17th ed. Ed. Janet Myers. Vienna, VA: PATC, 2008.
- USGS Quads: Harpers Ferry, Keedlesville, Middletown, and Myersville.

Hike southbound on Maryland's Blue Ridge, past Civil War relics, to a sublime, cliff-top view of one of the most historic towns in the United States: Harpers Ferry. A strategic point of great importance during the Civil War, this town is now a hub of outdoor recreation and one of the few through which the Appalachian Trail (AT) passes directly.

HIKE OVERVIEW

Taking advantage of Maryland's long and relatively flat ridges, you'll walk almost 25 moderate miles to enter Harpers Ferry—the "psychological halfway point" of the AT—much as a southbound thru-hiker would. Excellent overlooks abound on this route, including vistas from White Rocks, Weverton Cliffs, and Maryland Heights. This trip will also take you through countryside that served as a backdrop to some of the most important events of the Civil War; Harpers Ferry was taken eight times during the war and was the site of John Brown's famous raid—a bloody attempt to spark a slave revolt. You'll find a wealth of ruins and monuments on the trail to pique your curiosity and spark your imagination.

Although backpackers of all levels will enjoy this walk, beginner backpackers looking to expand their range will find this trip ideal. With lots of easy miles, only two climbs of note, and a single well-switchbacked descent, this is a fine choice for building up to more challenging trips.

HOW TO REACH THE TRAILHEAD

To Reach the Ending Trailhead. Head west from Frederick, Maryland, toward Harpers Ferry, West Virginia, on US 340. As you near Harpers Ferry, turn left on Keep Tryst Road, and then take a quick right on Sandy Hook Road. Pass the bridges to Harpers Ferry on your left, and soon, the steep wall of Maryland Heights on the right. Park your shuttle vehicles in the parking lots that serve the Maryland Heights trails, on the right (39° 19.7584' N, 77° 43.8984' W).

To Reach the Starting Trailhead. Retrace your route to US 340, take a right, and head east for about 0.5 mile. Then take the ramp for MD 67 toward Boonsboro. Proceed north about 13 miles with the ridge of the Maryland AT on your right. Turn left on South Main Street in downtown Boonsboro and take a right onto St. Paul Street, which becomes Boonsboro Mountain Road. Once you reach US 40, take a right. Cross I-70, and see the parking lot for the AT on the right (39° 32.1337' N, 77° 36.2386' W).

OVERNIGHT OPTIONS

Camping and campfires are not permitted on these sections of the AT, except at the following areas. Fortunately, these shelters and campgrounds are well spaced and offer you plenty of tenting opportunities. Backpackers on a three-day trip might start at I-70, spend one night at Rocky Run, and then a second night at Ed Garvey before arriving in Harpers Ferry on the third day, creating splits of 7, 8.5, and 9.2 miles, respectively.

Dahlgren Backpacker Campground (5.36/978/39° 28.886' N, 77° 37.146' W). Spot this campground on your right as you walk south from Turners Gap. Open all year, the campsite offers water, restrooms, and showers, though the restrooms close in winter.

Rocky Run Shelter (7.0/1,002/39° 27.656' N, 77° 37.852' W). This AT shelter is just west of the AT as you head south from Fox Gap. The shelter is strategically located before the climb up Lambs Knoll, and there is a good spring nearby and plenty of tent sites.

Crampton Gap Shelter (spur trail at 11.6/1,159, shelter at 39° 24.755' N, 77° 38.221' W). This is a fairly standard AT shelter that accommodates eight. There is a spring here, but it is described as sporadic and runs dry in summer.

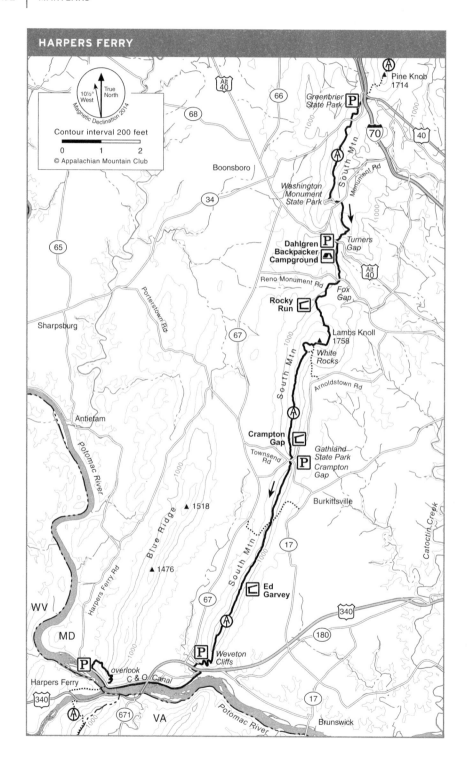

HARPERS FERRY

In a pinch, water can be had from a spigot in Gathland State Park, though it too is sometimes dry.

Ed Garvey Shelter (15.6/1,080/39° 21.589' N, 77° 39.703' W). Named after a former AT thru-hiker whose narrative of his trip inspired hikers in the 1970s and 1980s, the Ed Garvey Shelter is your must-have overnight spot for this trip. With a sleeping loft and balcony, Ed Garvey is a popular place to spend the night. It's often used by scout troops; however, plenty of tent sites are nearby. Check out those to the north of the shelter. Garvey's spring is reliable and vigorous, but it is a ways down the mountain to the east.

If you're interested in researching AT shelters before you leave home, check out whiteblaze.net, a website that, among other things, maintains threads on shelters up and down the AT. If you're doing this trip in warm weather, pay some attention to water, as sources do become rather sporadic between Rocky Run and Ed Garvey. Be sure to carry enough water to make it between these reliable springs.

HIKE DESCRIPTION

From the parking lot, follow the spur trail as it bends leftward and joins up with the AT on the north side of I-70. Cross the pedestrian bridge over the interstate, climb the stairs on the south side, and cross Boonsboro Mountain Road. For the next 0.9 mile, the trail passes along the eastern boundary of Greenbrier State Park. You'll leave the park behind you when you cross Boonsboro Mountain Road the second time.

After you cross a power cut, start a short, 250-foot climb to the intersection of the trail leading to the Washington Monument (3.1/1,536). This is another Washington Monument, quite different from its more famous cousin near the White House. First built in 1827, this monument was restored in the 1930s. Take the time to scope out the panorama of the surrounding countryside.

As you proceed south, the AT joins for a few hundred yards with the little trail that visitors use to reach the monument. Several placards describe George Washington's life. The trail soon reaches a parking lot, turns leftward, and crosses a few roads before it escapes to more isolated forest. A short descent takes you to Turners Gap, where the trail passes behind Dahlgren Chapel and then crosses US 40 Alt to the east of the Old South Mountain Inn (4.9/1,049). A parking lot is here for those using the AT.

South of Turners Gap, the AT shadows a couple of old roads, passes Dahlgren Backpacker Campground on the right (5.36/978), and soon arrives at Reno Monument Road at Fox Gap (6.1/1,053). This area saw especially heavy fighting during the Battle of South Mountain, and the monument on your left commemorates Major General Jesse Reno, a renegade Virginian who was mortally injured on this spot by a Confederate sharpshooter.

The AT bears rightward from this intersection and is fairly easy walking until after the spur trail to the Rocky Run Shelter, on your right (7.0/1,002). The trail then begins a 700-foot climb to the summit of Lambs Knoll, the toughest climb on this section. You'll cross a paved road and eventually spot a communication tower on your right as you near the top of the knoll (8.4/1,715).

The reward for this climb is the overlook from the cliffs at White Rocks (8.7/1,612), which allows you to look at the long line of the Blue Ridge marching southward to Virginia. From this angle, you'll easily appreciate the ruggedness of this terrain. Continue south along the AT. This quite typical Maryland ridgeline stretches for 4 miles before the trail reaches Crampton's Gap and Gathland State Park (12.0/927). Just before you begin the descent to the gap, spot a blue-blazed spur trail to the Crampton Gap Shelter on the left.

Crampton Gap also saw heavy fighting during the Civil War. On September 14, 1862, a Union force defeated a much smaller Confederate force in one of the many battles that raged around Harpers Ferry. The little park features a picnic pavilion, placards describing the battle, the remnants of an old stone barn, and a monument to Civil War newspaper correspondents. It's an excellent place to take a break and enjoy a sunny afternoon on your way south to the Ed Garvey Shelter. A vending machine and a pump that sometimes provides water are here. (The pump worked fine in February but is rumored to run dry in the hotter months.)

From Crampton Gap, the AT climbs 250 feet gently, but soon levels out to ridgeline walking for the 3.5 miles remaining to Ed Garvey. Throughout much of this portion of the walk, you'll have a rocky ridge on the east, with episodic views of Elk Ridge and the intervening valley to the west. Before long, the AT reaches a blue-blazed spur trail leading east to Ed Garvey and its excellent spring at the bottom of the hill (15.6/1,080).

After setting out from Ed Garvey, you have only 2.2 miles of walking before you reach Weverton Cliffs, one of the best views in Maryland. The trail becomes rockier as it heads south and reaches the sign marking the cliffs (17.8/846). Leave the AT and descend slabby terrain to catch the superb vista of the Potomac River flowing eastward from Harpers Ferry.

After taking in your fill of Weverton Cliffs, you'll have the sharpest descent of the trip ahead of you; the AT drops 600 feet down sixteen very-well-designed switchbacks. At the base of this descent, cross Weverton Road (18.4/370), then wander through some mixed terrain until you pass under a bridge for US 340, then over some railroad tracks. The AT turns right and begins heading west

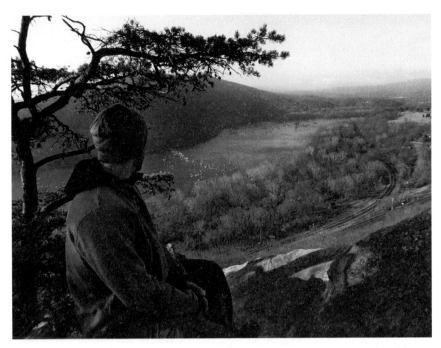

A hiker looks down on the Potomac as it flows from Harpers Ferry and past Weverton Cliffs.

along the C&O Canal (18.9/246). Enjoy perfectly flat walking along the canal towpath over the next 3 miles and views—of Harpers Ferry straight ahead, Loudoun Heights to the south, and Maryland Heights to the north—that get better as you proceed.

Upon reaching Harpers Ferry, the AT crosses the Potomac over a footbridge (21.5/259). If you like, feel free to explore the town, but your path actually continues a few tenths of a mile up the C&O towpath to where your vehicles are parked (22.0/278). Lock your packs in your vehicle and walk the trails of Maryland Heights. You'll have plenty of day-hiking company, but the sights really are incomparable.

Maryland Heights Combined Trail ascends fairly steeply from the road, bending around to the east and passing a naval gun emplacement on the right (22.2/684). The trails leading off to the left offer access to old Civil War ruins along the northern ridgeline (time permitting, walk these trails as well). For the main view of Harpers Ferry, however, continue east. The trail switchbacks down over about 0.4 mile and reaches a cliff overhanging the town and the confluence of the Shenandoah and Potomac rivers (23.4/628).

Among the grandest sights in the region, this overlook gives a keen sense of Harpers Ferry's importance to the transportation networks of the nineteenth century and its strategic significance. If you peer down at the three doors standing in a dismantled wall near the tip of the point, you can make out the ruins of the arsenal that John Brown seized on the night of October 16, 1859. An abolitionist, Brown believed that his raid would spark a slave revolt and that he would be able to escape into Virginia, freeing slaves as he went. Instead, he was cornered in the arsenal, and a small unit of U.S. Marines, under the command of Robert E. Lee and J.E.B. Stuart, put down the revolt. Brown was hanged for treason on December 2, 1859. His last words: "I, John Brown, am now quite certain that the crimes of this guilty land can never be purged away but with blood."

Continue exploring the ruins up high, or head for the town itself. Returning directly to your vehicle completes the 24.7-mile trip.

OTHER OPTIONS

Easy accessibility to the AT allows plenty of options for shortening this trip to take on fewer miles. Instead of starting at I-70, use Turners Gap or Gathland State Park as starting places. Similarly, by parking a vehicle at the base of Weverton Cliffs, you shave off the 4.3 miles of walking along the C&O Canal into Harpers Ferry. These last miles, however, are worth keeping if you can; the walk along the canal is peaceful and the trip to Maryland Heights offers the best scenery along the route.

NEARBY

The town of Harpers Ferry is a fascinating place to visit, and a historical tour of the city is always in order. Several bars and restaurants cater to tourists, and there is an outfitters shop that is well known to those who have walked the AT. Harpers Ferry is also the home of the Appalachian Trail Conservancy and the AT Visitor Center at 799 W. Washington Street. If you do this trip during summer, end it with a cooling float down the Potomac River. Numerous tubing and rafting outfitters surround the town.

ADDITIONAL INFORMATION

For more information, contact the Appalachian Trail Conservancy, 304-535-6331, info@appalachiantrail.org; PATC, 703-242-0315; or the South Mountain Recreation Area, 301-791-4656.

TRIP 27
ON THE ROCKS

Location: Gambrill State Park, Maryland
Highlights: Views from Annapolis Rock, Black Rock, Raven Rock, Hog Rock, Chimney Rock, and Cat Rock
Distance: 47.7 miles one-way
Total Elevation Gain/Loss: 9,047 feet/8,918 feet
Trip Length: 3–6 days
Difficulty: Strenuous
Recommended Maps and Other Resources:
- *PATC, Maps 5 and 6: Appalachian Trail across Maryland and the Entire Catoctin Trail*, 18th edition, 2009.
- National Park Service, "Catoctin Mountain Map," nps.gov/cato.
- Gambrill State Park, "Gambrill State Park Features and Trail System," dnr.maryland.gov/publiclands/maps/gambrillmap.html.
- Hiking Upward, "Catoctin Trail Hike," hikingupward.com/OMH/CatoctinTrail.
- USGS Quads: Blue Ridge, Catoctin Furnace, Frederick, Myersville, and Smithsburg.

While local day-hikers are familiar with many of the highlights of this trip, few link up the Appalachian Trail (AT) with Catoctin Trail (CT) for a backpacking trip of this level of ambition and grandeur—all within an hour's drive from the Baltimore–DC metropolitan area. The CT varies from being extremely frequently traveled by day-hikers to rarely being visited in its wilder stretches. Along the way, you'll reel off one big view of the Maryland Blue Ridge after another. You'll see Annapolis Rock and Ravens Rock from the AT, and you'll summit Chimney Rock, Wolf Rock, and Cat Rock. Keep in mind, too, that the hike across Maryland is about 40 miles long; this route will take you very near to the big 5-0.

HIKE OVERVIEW

If you lay out a topographic map of Maryland's Blue Ridge Mountains, your eye will quickly recognize how the long line of the AT—running straight north from Harpers Ferry, West Virginia, to Pen Mar, Maryland—all but intersects the line of the CT, which snakes its way southeast from Raven Rock Road. Your map is just begging you to join up these trails; you know you can't resist this challenge! Admittedly, you'll need 2.4 miles of uninspiring road walking to link up the two trails, but that's a small price to pay to join up two of Maryland's best hiking routes into a single trip. Big views are a staple of the Maryland AT's long and relatively level ridgelines; in contrast, the CT requires a few detours to reach some of the best hiking sights in the state—Cunningham Falls, Hog Rock, Wolf Rock, Chimney Rock, and Cat Rock.

HOW TO REACH THE TRAILHEAD

The easiest parking arrangement for this route is a horseshoe shuttle in which you park two vehicles relatively close together but at different trailhead parking lots. In this case, you'll leave your anchor vehicle at the Gambrill State Park trailhead for the CT, and the other at the AT parking lot just off I-70, near Annapolis Rocks. To leave a vehicle overnight in the Gambrill State Park parking lot, you'll need to contact the rangers there at 301-271-7574. Call for permission a few days ahead.

Both trailheads are easy to reach, especially from the Baltimore–Washington, D.C. area. From Frederick, Maryland, head west on US 40. After about 5 miles, turn right, first onto Five Forks Road, and then continue onto Gambrill Park Road. The parking lot for the CT (the ending trailhead) is on the right (39° 27.733' N, 77° 29.473' W). Leave a vehicle there and return to US 40. Continue west for roughly 10 miles until you see the parking lot for the AT on the left. Park here (39° 32.129' N, 77° 36.237' W).

OVERNIGHT OPTIONS

There are a number of excellent camping spots along the AT in Maryland. While the CT also passes by several established campgrounds, they are open only during the warmer months, so their availability will influence when you can walk this trip. Note that the entire stretch of the CT from the Manor Area Campground to Gambrill State Park does not permit backcountry camping, so plan to cross this approximately 15-mile stretch in a single day. If that's more than you're willing to bite off, shorten this leg by 5 miles by placing your anchor vehicle at Hamburg Road rather than at the CT trailhead (see Other Options).

Annapolis Rock Campsite (2.56/1,686/39° 33.527' N, 77° 35.871' W). Just a few feet from Annapolis Rock, you'll spot several tent pads for backcountry camping. This campsite makes a great option if you're planning to arrive at the trailhead late and want to walk just a few miles before making camp. There is a privy, a picnic table, and a spring. Campfires are prohibited.

ANNAPOLIS ROCK

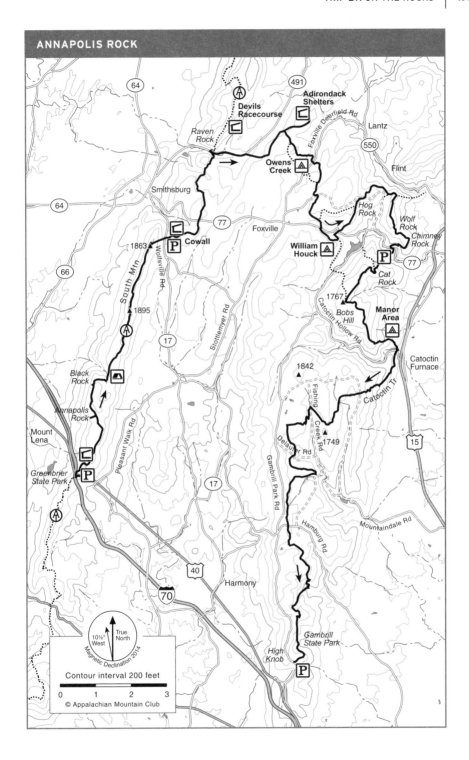

64

491

**Devils
Racecourse**

**Adirondack
Shelters**

Raven
Rock

550

Lantz

**Owens
Creek**

Flint

Smithsburg

64

77

Foxville

Hog
Rock

Wolf
Rock

Chimney
Rock

1863

Cowall

**William
Houck**

P

77

South Mtn

Woltsville Rd

66

Cat
Rock

1895

Stottlemyer Rd

17

1767

Bobs
Hill

Catoctin Hollow Rd

**Manor
Area**

Catoctin Furnace

Black
Rock

1842

Catoctin Tr

Annapolis
Rock

Pleasant Walk Rd

Fishing Creek Rd

1749

15

Mount
Lena

P

Delauter Rd

Gambrill Park Rd

**Greenbrier
State Park**

17

Hamburg Rd

Mountaindale Rd

40

70

Harmony

Gambrill
State Park

High
Knob

P

10½°
West

True
North

Magnetic Declination 2014

Contour interval 200 feet

0   1   2   3

© Appalachian Mountain Club

Cowall Shelter (8.8/1,366/39° 37.861′ N, 77° 33.34′ W). A very nice, new shelter that may fit in well with your hike itinerary. Water is available nearby, and there are tent pads in the vicinity.

Devil's Racecourse Shelter (leave route at 12.1/1,061; shelter is 1 mile north on the AT, and 0.1 miles off the trail on a spur to the left) Just north of Raven Rock Road is the new (and quite comfortable) Devil's Racecourse Shelter (about 1.1 miles away from MD 491). If you reach Raven Rock Road late in the day, staying here is a good option.

Mount Zion Road Adirondacks Shelters (15.8/1,454/39° 40.635′ N, 77° 29.082′ W). After you reach the northernmost trailhead for the CT (14.8/1,567), turn north and walk about 1 mile. A broad, unblazed trail will take you to the Adirondacks Shelters. Each of these two shelters can accommodate five people, but you must reserve them either at the Catoctin Mountain Visitor Center or online at nps.gov/cato/planyourvisit/adiron.htm. A privy is near the shelters, and there are fire pits. Bring your own water, however, as the nearby stream was little more than a trickle when I visited. Tent camping is not permitted in the vicinity of these shelters.

Owens Creek Campground (18/1,237/39° 39.583′ N, 77° 29.051′ W). Not far from the northern end of the CT, Owens Creek Campground offers tent camping sites for $20 per night. The sites are available on a first-come, first-served basis. There are two "comfort stations," one of which has hot showers. Open from May through November.

Manor Area Campground (32.2/622/39° 35.242′ N, 77° 26.164′ W). Open from April through November, this established campsite offers tent sites, fire rings, and a bathhouse. For a fee ranging from $11.75 to $61.75, depending on the season and the type of site, you can spend the night here and get an early jump on the last 15 miles of the walk to Gambrill State Park. You'll see the spur trail for this campsite on the left as you reach the bottom of Bobs Hill.

HIKE DESCRIPTION

From the back of the AT's parking lot on US 40, a spur trail leads in short order to the footbridge spanning I-70. You're headed north, so don't cross the interstate. Take a hard right, follow the trail along I-70, and begin the gently graded climb up to Annapolis Rock.

Over the next 2.25 miles, you'll climb about 500 feet, passing a blue-blazed trail leading left to Pine Knob Shelter after about a half-mile. Nearly 2.5 miles from the trailhead, a westward spur trail leads to the cliffs of Annapolis Rock (2.48/1,646). It's about 0.2 mile to the view, but well worth it, as this is one of the better views along the Maryland AT.

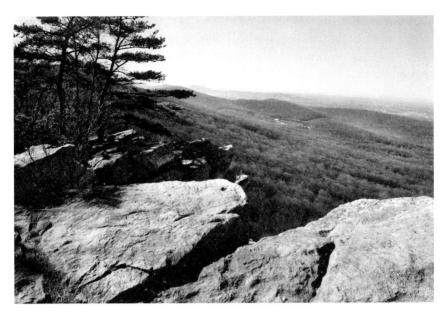

On a clear day, Annapolis Rock offers impressive westward views.

Return to the AT, and head north. You'll rack up easy miles along the rela-tively flat ridgeline, passing rocky promontories that offer views to the east and the west. You'll visit Black Rock (3.76/1,794) and drop down to the Pogo Memorial Campsite (named after a member of the Mountain Club of Mary-land, Walter "Pogo" Rheinheimer, Jr.). If you're in need of water, a spring at the Pogo campsite is fairly reliable (4.32/1,519). After the campsite, the trail climbs back up to a ridgeline that starts to become rockier. The AT eventually climbs steeply to crest the ridge, then switchbacks down to Wolfsville Road/MD 17, about 500 feet below (8.69/1,333). Just on the far side of the road, a blue-blazed trail leads to a useful parking lot, but the AT continues north, passing a creek, and then tent sites and the well-constructed Cowall Shelter (8.8/1,366). There is also a spring near this shelter.

The trail crosses a power cut and continues to climb steeply, eventually passing through meadows as it turns left and reaches Foxsville Road/MD 77 (10/1,594). North of the road, it passes through a few agricultural fields, and then begins a steady descent toward Warner Gap Road (11.6/1,146). Just be-fore the gravel road, the trail crosses a stream on a rather peculiar "bridge to nowhere." It almost gets you all the way across the creek, but where would be the challenge in that?

Turn left on Warner Hollow Road, and then quickly leave the road on the right. Climb up and over the right shoulder of Buzzard Knob, jump over an ancient stone wall, then descend about 300 feet to cross Little Antietam Creek (12.4/1,074). At Raven Rock Road/MD 491, your route diverges from the AT, but if you have time, take a short detour to the sharp cliffs of Devil's Race-course by continuing north for 0.2 mile and doubling back. The Raven Rock shelter north of the road is a good overnight option if you've reached this point at the end of the day.

From the intersection of the AT and Raven Rock Road, the trailhead for the CT is a regrettable 2.4 miles of road walking away. Start by walking eastward on the wide shoulder of Raven Rock Road. As the road bends to the north, turn right on Hells Delight Road (no kidding) and climb until it intersects with Quirauk School Road. Turn left and proceed slightly downhill until you reach an awkward intersection with Mount Zion Road, which sneaks in on the left. You'll be able to see the white Mount Zion United Methodist Church ahead on the left. The trailhead for the CT is directly across from the church (14.8/1,567).

If you're making for the Adirondacks Shelters in the north, take a left at the fork in the trail just past the trailhead and follow the road grade about 1 mile, past some old stone fences on the left. Eventually, you'll spot the shelter on the left (15.8/1,454). (Note: Subsequent mile markers assume you visited the shelters. If you didn't, you can subtract 2 miles.) If you're ready to begin your southward trek on the CT, take the right at the fork in the road. Soon enough, you'll start spotting the blue blazes of the CT.

Your first few miles along the CT will be a gradual descent toward Owens Creek and Foxville Road/MD 77. The CT crosses both where the road enters the Owens Creek Campground (18/1,234). From here, the trail climbs a bit, follows an old forest road closely, and at times walks along it. Away on your left is Camp David—not a good spot to stray from the trail. The trail descends steadily, crosses MD 77 (20.6/1,363), climbs steeply up the far side, and then traverses some rocky, uneven ground before it reaches an intersection with the trail to Cunningham Falls.

Here the CT heads southeasterly, but you'll be making a northerly grand detour to take in all the best sights of Catoctin Mountain Park. (Note that trails in the park are not blazed like the CT or the AT. They are, however, well signed and easy to follow.) Turn left and walk about 200 feet down to Big Hunting Creek and Cunningham Falls (21.4/1,183). This picturesque 78-foot-tall cascade is the largest waterfall in Maryland. You'll need to reach the second boardwalk north of the creek and head to MD 77—you'll be able to spot a trail on the opposite side of the road. Continue 500 feet up the trail marked for Hog Rock (1,610).

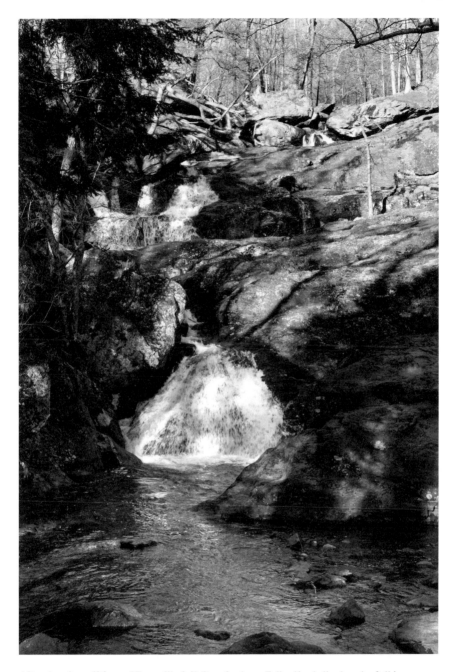

After turning off from CT, you'll visit Cunningham Falls, the tallest waterfall in Maryland.

Hog Rock rewards you with an eastward panorama of the next few hours of your journey (22.6/1,612). Your route will swing out to the left, offering northerly views. Then the trail marches along the long arm of the ridge you see in front of you, and it will pass Wolf Rock and Chimney Rock before descending to the gap at MD 77 and climbing up to the ridgeline on your right to Cat Rock and Bobs Hill beyond it.

Pass by side trails for Hog Rock Nature Trail, then cross Park Central Road, where there is a parking lot and a toilet. A quick climb takes you to the Blue Ridge Summit Overlook (23.4/1,520). The trail then descends a bit and traverses woodlands with partial views on your left.

When you reach a four-way intersection, bear left and climb again to a view at Thurmont Vista (24.3/1,499). In about 1 mile, the trail arrives at Wolf Rock, where side trails will take you on a rocky spine along which you may scramble, and finally to Chimney Rock (25.8/1,419), a prow-like cliff looking out over eastern Maryland. I highly recommend that you climb out on the rocks (beware the fissures!) and enjoy lunch or a snack at this fine vista.

When you're ready to move on, return from Chimney Rock and follow the trail to the right as it sweeps around the high point. The trail soon splits again. Follow the rightward trail toward the park headquarters. This descent is steep and rocky before the trail reaches the headquarters building (26.9/828) and crosses MD 77. Look across to the road to the left, and you'll see the trailhead for Cat Rock (the trail is yellow blazed). Water is readily available here.

The climb up to Cat Rock is challenging, perhaps the toughest climb on this trip. In about 1.3 miles, you'll ascend about 800 feet at a steady grade. After you pass a power cut, a spur trail leads to Cat Rock itself, where you can scramble up to the summit (28.2/1,562). Follow the yellow-blazed trail south; it stays fairly level until it rejoins the CT. From the juncture with the blue-blazed the CT (29.7/1,743), turn left and walk eastward along the broad back of Bobs Hill. Largely level walking will eventually take you to a leftward spur trail to the summit of the hill (30.3/1,765), where a sharp series of slabs invites you to enjoy the big views of Maryland farmlands.

The descent off Bobs Hill is surprising. Where, exactly, does a 1,200-foot descent come from in the mountains of Maryland? The trail switchbacks at an uncomfortable grade, passes a turnoff for the Manor Area Campground on the left, and then becomes a bit sketchy as it dips down to Hunting Creek (32.3/563). Crossing Hunting Creek is no easy rock hop. I walked straight across (getting wet below the knees), but others in my party contrived to get across dry. If it looks at all high, walk out to US 15 and use the bridge to cross.

From Hunting Creek to Hamburg Road is perhaps the wildest bit of walking on this trip. While the CT is usually fairly well maintained and blazed, in stretches the blazes can become less frequent, the trail less maintained, the route somewhat cryptic. Climb from Hunting Creek to Catoctin Hollow Road, and then reascend a steady grade to the ridgeline. The forest along the trail shows signs of having recently been devastated by a catastrophic weather event, perhaps the derecho of 2012. While the trail maintenance crews have been busy with their chainsaws, some blowdowns may still be impassable without detours.

After a few switchbacks toward the top, the trail crests at a rocky overlook with views to the east (34.4/1,390). The walking becomes easier as you enter the City of Frederick Municipal Forest. You'll cross several roads, pass a few ponds, and then reach Fishing Creek Road and Steep Creek (36.8/1,488). A few rock hops across the branches of this little creek and you'll be climbing from the little basin. The trail here has been rerouted, and you'll find the path rather serpentine. Eventually the trail will bend leftward and become extremely eroded before it reaches a pond (with a rope swing, if you dare!). The trail turns right and soon passes Delauter Road (39.2/1,455). The CT crosses the road and seems almost to run through a resident's backyard before regaining the forest.

Easy walking for about 3 miles takes you south to Hamburg Road—you'll notice the sharp westward bend in the trail visible on the PATC map. When you reach a pond, you may choose to walk around it if you like. There are at least two trails leading from this pond to Hamburg Road—one is blazed blue, the other is not, but both are well maintained and lead more or less due south to the parking lot on Hamburg Road (42.3/1,619).

You have just over 5 miles remaining until the end of the trail. As you head to Gambrill State Park, you'll notice that the trail is not always blazed as well as you might like, and some blue blazes are even blacked out. The trail goes on, however, and a leftward bend takes you down a steep slope into a creek basin that marks the border of the park (44.9/916). Cross the creek several times during the steep climb up this pretty little hollow. Do be alert, however, as the trail will veer off to the left toward the top of the climb. The CT emerges briefly onto a forest road (46/1,491), where you'll take a right, but then take a left onto a trail that is now blazed blue and yellow (you'll see that there are now trail maps and signs at many intersections).

Gambrill State Park has a quite a few little trails, all of which will eventually get you to your vehicle. If you are a purist, stay on the blue-blazed CT as it fraternizes with the yellow and then the green and the black trails. The CT will give you another dip and a climb, but what does that matter after almost 50 miles? The yellow-blazed trail will take you to the park's best vistas, or you can explore as you like until it's time to end your journey at the trailhead where all trails meet (47.7/1,349).

OTHER OPTIONS

Obviously, with the AT and its many points of access, you have options for lengthening or abridging this trip. Most notably, you could add miles by starting at Turners Gap instead of I-70, which would add about 5 miles, or even starting all the way at the base of Weverton Cliffs, which would add about 19 miles. If you choose to start that close to Harpers Ferry, you'll just be a few miles from hiking all the way across Maryland. An out-and-back to Pen-Mar (the Pennsylvania border and the Mason-Dixon Line) from the Raven Rock Shelter is a possibility.

Conversely, you could shorten the trip by placing your anchor vehicle at Hamburg Road rather than Gambrill State Park, trimming 5 miles from the end of the hike. Close study of the maps could yield a number of other options, including ideas for section-hiking the trip over a few weekends.

NEARBY

Of course, Frederick, Maryland, is very close and offers you all the trappings of civilization. Visit downtown, and as you'll be impressed by the number and quality of eateries. It's an ideal watering hole after a few days on the trail.

ADDITIONAL INFORMATION

If you're looking for additional information, you may contact PATC at 703-242-0315 or at patc.net. Cunningham Falls State Park and Gambrill State Park can be reached at 301-271-7574 or online at dnr.state.md.us. Finally, the Catoctin Mountain Park's phone number is 301-663-9388, and its website is nps.gov/cato/.

6

NEW JERSEY AND DELAWARE

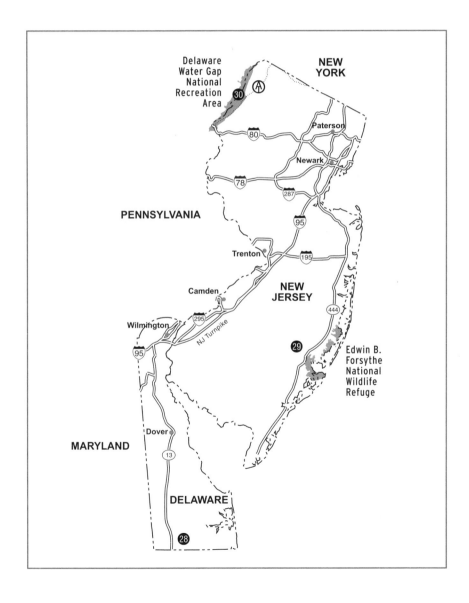

TRIP 28
BEWARE THE PIRANHA-CONDA!

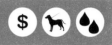

Location: Trap Pond State Park, Delaware
Highlights: Freshwater wetlands, abundant wildlife, the northernmost baldcypress trees in the United States
Distance: 6.81 miles round-trip
Total Elevation Gain/Loss: 192 feet gain/192 feet loss
Trip Length: 2 days
Difficulty: Easy
Recommended Maps and Other Resources:
- Delaware State Parks, *Trap Pond State Park*, 2009. destateparks.com/downloads/maps/trap-pond/trap-pond-2009.pdf.
- USGS Quad: Trap Pond.

Trap Pond is the last remaining vestige of the freshwater wetlands that once covered this portion of Delaware and Maryland. As you hike its trails and paddle its waterways, you'll be exploring a rich ecosystem that is unique in the Mid-Atlantic. Keep your eyes peeled, as the park is rich in all manner of wildlife; bird watchers especially enjoy this environment as herons, owls, hummingbirds, and even the occasional bald eagle call this pond home. You'll find the second-growth baldcypress trees and the swamps they inhabit a fascinating change of pace from the mountains, rivers, and forests we backpackers usually enjoy.

HIKE OVERVIEW

Trap Pond was formed when loggers dammed the creek to power a sawmill that turned many of the old-growth trees into lumber. Paradoxically, the pond has now become a haven for second-growth baldcypress trees and for the wildlife that depends on this unique ecosystem. While the experience of trekking around Trap Pond is certainly more frontcountry than backcountry, the park provides a new backpacker with an excellent opportunity for a first overnight foray. The gentleness of the terrain and the comparative ease of the hiking will mean that you'll be able to try out your various pieces of equipment and build skill, without worrying much if things don't go exactly as planned. And while the hiking is not difficult, almost 7 miles of walking will give you a

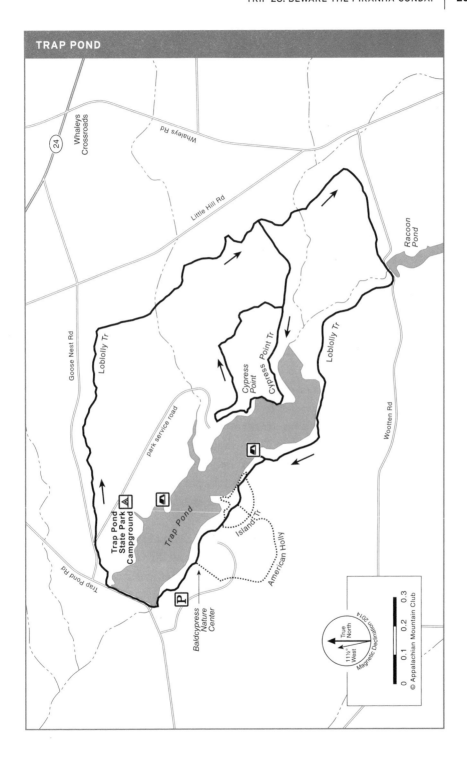

TRAP POND

24
Whaleys Crossroads
Whaleys Rd
Little Hill Rd
Racoon Pond
Goose Nest Rd
Loblolly Tr
Cypress Point
Cypress Point Tr
Loblolly Tr
Wootten Rd
Park service road
Trap Pond State Park Campground
Trap Pond
Island Tr
American Holly
Trap Pond Rd
Baldcypress Nature Center
True North
11½° West
Magnetic Declination 2014
0   0.1   0.2   0.3
© Appalachian Mountain Club

chance to evaluate how well that fully loaded pack really feels or if those boots actually fit.

This route follows a 6.8-mile circumnavigation of the park, primarily on Loblolly Trail. As written, the trip assumes you'll vehicle-camp in the family campground, but you can also walk into one of the primitive sites and join up with the described loop easily enough. Either way, practice setting up and striking camp, as if you were in the backcountry.

HOW TO REACH THE TRAILHEAD

From Annapolis and the Chesapeake Bay Bridge, drive east on US 50 for about 20 miles. Turn left onto MD 404 and follow it for 24 miles, at which point it will enter Delaware. Six miles into the state, turn left on DE 404 E/Newton Road and follow it for 2 miles. Then turn right onto DE 404/US 13 and take it south for almost 15 miles. In Laurel, Delaware, turn left onto DE 24 and drive east about 5 miles. Turn right onto Trap Pond Road. Take a left on Goose Nest Road and follow the signs to the campground (38° 31.8417' N, 75° 28.5514' W).

OVERNIGHT OPTIONS

Trap Pond State Park offers you a number of overnight options. A fee is associated with each; residents of Delaware receive a discount.

Family Camping on the North Shore (0.0/37/38° 31.775' N, 75° 28.598' W). All the pleasure of vehicle camping, complete with showers, toilets, and a camp store. Rates range from $25 to $30/per night.

Primitive Camping along Trap Pond (5.52/36/38° 31.354' N, 75° 28.327' W). Call to inquire about reserving these attractive tenting sites, some of which include pavilions and privies. Rates range from $20 to $30/per night. The walk is short, and the views are beautiful.

The park also has a number of yurts and cabins that you may inquire about renting. The rates run up to $61 a night. To contact the park directly, call 302-875-2392; to make overnight reservations, call 877-921-8151 or visit delawarestateparks.reserveamerica.com/.

HIKE DESCRIPTION

For this trip, you'll be walking a loop around Trap Pond, mainly on the Loblolly Trail. From the campground entrance (at the 10 o'clock poisiton), begin walking clockwise along Loblolly Trail. The terrain is flat, the trail paved, the walking smooth and even, so you should find this first stretch of the trail easy going as you round the park's north side. You'll pass a number of swamps and waterways. Keep your eye out for reptiles and amphibians. On my trip,

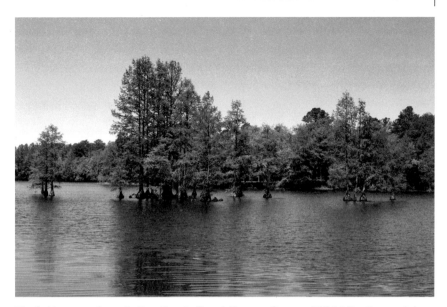

The baldcypress trees in Trap Pond offer visitors a glimpse of Mid-Atlantic coastal wetlands before settlers tamed these lands.

I spotted no fewer than three black snakes (two of whom were locked in an amorous embrace), and dozens of bullfrogs sang to me.

When you reach the intersection with the unnamed multiuse trail (1.53/40) at the 3 o'clock position, you'll walk a quick out-and-back to get a better look at the swamps and the baldcypress trees. Hang a right and follow the signs for Cypress Point. You'll walk along a broad path for about a half-mile, and then you'll encounter Cypress Point Trail, which crosses your path (2.06/40). Take a left on this path. The trail will become more of a footpath and the footing will become a bit more uneven. Be sure to explore the various spur trails leading to the pond. Eventually, Cypress Point Trail will come to a trailhead (2.58/37), then turn back to the east. Be sure to stay on the trail, as there's a disc golf trail that confuses things a bit. Turn left and follow it back to Loblolly Trail (3.75/40). You've returned to the 3 o'clock position on your loop.

Take a right. You'll pass over a few boardwalks with interesting views of the swamps below (4.0/42) before the trail turns right just shy of Wootten Road (4.15/42), at about 5 o'clock. It will join up with the road, cross Raccoon Pond, and then turn right to begin heading north (4.6/38). The Loblolly Trail follows the pond's shoreline northwesterly for about 1.75 miles along a gravel path. Again, the best views are to be had by exploring the spur trails to the right. You'll pass intersections for Island Trail and then reach the developed area around Baldcypress Nature Center (6.10/35) at 9 o'clock.

Continue to follow Loblolly Trail as it passes the boat house and turns right over a bridge for Trap Pond Road (6.36/34). An informative placard describes how Trap Pond was created to serve the various mills that used to operate here. On the far side of the pond, take a right at the boat launch and pass to the left of the family campground (6.56/34). You'll soon return to the campground's entrance (6.81/37).

OTHER OPTIONS

Because Trap Pond itself is rather self-contained, there aren't many opportunities to add miles on foot. The park, however, rents a variety of boats, including kayaks and canoes. Exploring the pond and swamps by water, along one of the established canoe trails, will allow you to add another dimension to your trip.

NEARBY

There is no shortage of local businesses in Laurel and Seaford, Delaware. Drive a little farther south on US 13 to reach Salisbury, Maryland, which is the nearest large town.

ADDITIONAL INFORMATION

For more information, visit Trap Pond State Park's website at destateparks .com/park/trap-pond/ or call 302-875-5153.

TRIP 29
THE DEVIL WENT DOWN TO JERSEY

Location: Pinelands National Reserve, New Jersey
Highlights: Rare glimpse of an undeveloped Atlantic coastal forest, unique ecosystem with unusual plants and animals
Distance: 21.3 miles one-way
Total Elevation Gain/Loss: 520 feet gain/536 feet loss
Trip Length: 2–3 days
Difficulty: Easy
Recommended Maps and Other Resources:
- *BATONA Trail*, New Jersey State Park Service, 2010. state.nj.us/dep/parksandforests/parks/docs/batona14web.pdf.
- *Bass River State Forest Hiking Trails*, New Jersey State Park Service, 2008. state.nj.us/dep/parksandforests/parks/docs/Bass%20River%20Trail%20Map.pdf. Detailed map of Lake Absegami area.
- USGS Quads: Oswego Lake, New Gretna, Jenkins, and Green Bank.

Located in the heart of one of the most urbanized areas of the United States, the Pine Barrens is a 1.1-million-acre area of Atlantic coast that remains almost entirely undeveloped. Though many settlements rose and fell during this region's long history, few stand now as anything other than desolate ghost towns. For hikers, the backbone of this area is the BAck TO NAture Trail (or BATONA), which traces a 50-mile path through this wild country. Though it is unlikely that you'll catch a glimpse of the fabled Jersey Devil, you're almost certain to cross paths with a number of unusual reptiles, amphibians, orchids, and carnivorous plants.

HIKE OVERVIEW

With essentially no elevation change and exceedingly gentle footing, this trip is suitable for new backpackers who want to practice, build skill with their equipment, and learn what the Pine Barrens are all about. And you can't ask for a more centrally located wilderness.

This trip is designed for new backpackers wishing to spend a weekend getting a taste of BATONA. After setting up a vehicle shuttle on Friday, you'd arrive at Lake Absegami, where you could choose to stretch your legs with a 3.9-mile loop from the South Shore Campsite at Bass River State Park.

Saturday morning, depart for 10.4 miles of flat walking along BATONA (plus a road or two to reach Godfrey Bridge Family Camp), and then, on day three, 10.4 more miles to finish up at Batsto. You'll come away with a much sharper understanding of backpacking and a keener appreciation of this unique ecosystem.

A word to the wise, however. Visit the Pine Barrens in cooler months, well before the insects have hatched. This area can become quite oppressive in the heat and can serve as a breeding ground for a wide variety of hostile insects, including ticks and chiggers. You should always take precautions to keep the bugs away.

HOW TO REACH THE TRAILHEAD

To Reach the Ending Trailhead. From I-295 in New Jersey, just across the Delaware River from Philadelphia, take US 30 east for about 23 miles. Outside of Hammonton, New Jersey, take a left onto CR 542. As you drive east, look for the sign indicating Batsto Village. From the north, take the New Jersey Turnpike and take exit 7 to US 206 south. Drive 33 miles, then take lefts on Airport Road and CR 542 to reach Batsto Village. Pull in and leave one vehicle here to anchor your shuttle (39° 38.676' N, 74° 38.816' W).

To Reach the Starting Trailhead. Continue driving east on CR 542. Continue on to CR 653, and then turn left into the Bass River State Forest, not far from the Garden State Parkway. Follow the signs to the campground (39° 37.270' N, 74° 25.416' W).

OVERNIGHT OPTIONS

Camping along BATONA is only allowed at established campsites, so plan to stay at Lake Absegami Camp Friday night and Godfrey Bridge Saturday. Your end-point is Batsto, so you can also consider spending the night at the Button Wood Hill Camp, but you would only spend the night there if you wished to spend an extra night on the trail. Note that these campsites are not located on BATONA itself.

South Shore 39° 37.596' N, 74° 25.162' W). Located very near the trailhead, this campground in Bass River State Park offers a wide variety of campsites, lean-tos, shelters, and cabins. You won't find solitude or silence here, but the campground does offer plenty of conveniences such as bathrooms, fire rings, showers, and laundry facilities. Plan on camping here for the first night of a three-day trip and setting out on BATONA on day two. Fees vary based on the site you choose, but the basic site is $20 for New Jersey residents and $25 for others.

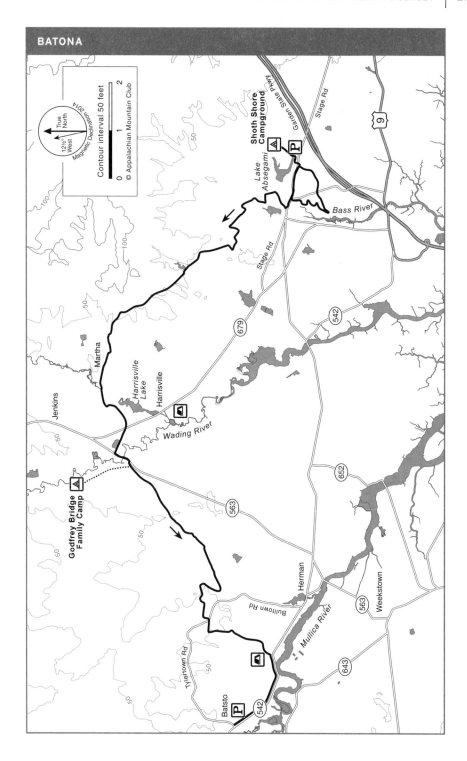

BATONA

Contour interval 50 feet

© Appalachian Mountain Club

True North

12½° West

Magnetic Declination 2014

Shoth Shore Campground

Garden State Pkwy

Stage Rd

US 9

Lake Absegami

Bass River

Stage Rd

679

542

Martha

Harrisville Lake

Harrisville

Wading River

Jenkins

Godfrey Bridge Family Camp

563

652

Herman

Bulltown Rd

563

Weekstown

Mullica River

Tylertown Rd

Batsto

542

643

Godfrey Bridge Family Camp (leave route at 14.4, campground at 39° 41.389' N, 74° 32.837' W). Though off the trail a few miles, this campground offers a fair number of amenities. You may reach it from BATONA by leaving the trail at CR 563, walking north about 1.8 miles, and then taking a left on Godfrey Bridge Road and walking 1.2 miles to the campsite. With a number of sites, potable water, fire rings, picnic tables, and pit toilets, this is an attractive place to spend the night. It's $3 per person per night for New Jersey residents; $5 per person per night for others.

Buttonwood Hill Camp (21.3/39° 37.744' N, 74° 37.067' W). Located in Wharton State Forest right along CR 542, this much more primitive campsite offers space for up to five groups of six. The site includes a pit toilet, but potable water is available only seasonally at Crowleys Landing, about a quarter-mile to the south. It's $3 per person per night for New Jersey residents; $5 per person per night for others. Reach this site by leaving BATONA at the signed intersection, where blue blazes will lead you southward (19.8). The campsite is 1.5 miles farther along.

All these sites require reservations through ReserveAmerica.com. To avoid extra online fees, call ReserveAmerica at 877-444-6777.

HIKE DESCRIPTION

After camping Friday evening at the near Lake Abesgami, go for a quick hike to stretch your legs and get a sense for the environment. Walk toward the office for Bass River State Park, where all the trails (blazed with different colors) come together. Look for a pink-blazed loop. Be careful to distinguish the pink blazes from those for the Plum Trail, which is blazed with a very similar color. Some of the blazes have even faded to white, but rangers have written in the word "pink" or "plum" on many of them.

Initially, follow a combined pink- and red-blazed trail along the southern bank of the lake. Soon the pink trail crosses Stage Road and follows it on the left for about 0.7 mile. It then crosses East Green Bush Road (1.48) and winds south through cedar swamps, pine plantations, and some pine and oak forest. It turns eastward, recrosses the road (3.1), and then follows forest trails as it continues east and then north. It crosses the road (3.89) and passes back by the state park office to your campsite.

Saturday morning, when you're ready to begin your trek on BATONA, begin by walking along the pink-blazed trail as it follows Stage Road. Initially, this is ground you walked the previous day. Where the pink blazes turns south, however, continue along Stage Road for about 1,200 feet more. On the right, you should spot BATONA's trailhead (4.86), which is well marked. Instead of

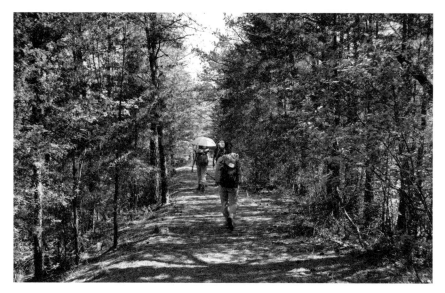

In cool weather, you will enjoy easy walking along the wide, flat trails of the Pine Barrens.

continuing directly westward, as the map indicates, there is a reroute, which takes you north and westward. BATONA is well blazed, so that should make things easier. You have about 7.7 miles to walk to reach Martha Bridge.

Walk northward along Dan Bridge Road, bearing northeast. Keep your eyes peeled, however, as BATONA's pink blazes will soon lead off to the west (left) at a sharp angle (5.35). At this point, the trail takes you into the barrens. Immediately, you'll start to appreciate the unique experience of walking in this unusual coastal Atlantic forest—the footway is smooth, wide, and sandy, and usually covered in pine needles. This sandy, nutrient-poor soil accounts for the lack of development on this coastal plain. Although it was too poor for agriculture, it is a haven for the varieties of pine trees you see around you, including the ubiquitous pitch pines, which depend on fire to reproduce.

Pass a number of bogs, ponds, and canals before the trail reaches Martha Bridge, a dilapidated structure spanning a tea-colored stream (12.5). Refill your bottles here and, time permitting, soak in the cooling waters of the creek. The trail will hustle you on, crossing first CR 689 (13.8) and meeting CR 563 (14.4). At this second road, BATONA turns left and heads south along its eastern shoulder. If you're headed for the Godfrey Bridge Family Camp, turn north here instead. Walk about 3 miles to reach this camp.

Sunday morning, return to where BATONA intersects CR 563. The trail follows CR 563 about 0.3 mile to the south, then it turns right, crosses the road, and plunges once again into the pinelands (14.7). Over the next 7 miles, the trail occasionally becomes narrower, with vegetation closing in on the path. After crossing Washington Road (16.5), the trail reaches an intersection marked with signs pointing the way to the Buttonwood Hill Campsite (19.8). The pink blazes of the BATONA continue to head west; follow the blue blazes south instead.

In 1.5 miles, the blue-blazed trail arrives at the campsite, CR 542, and your vehicle (21.3).

About 3.4 miles further along, you will arrive at the village of Batsto, where your vehicles await (23.2).

OTHER OPTIONS
It is possible to plan backpacking trips of varying lengths along BATONA by making use of the numerous spots where the trail crosses a road. One could, in this manner, section-hike the trail, walking from Bass River State Park to Batsto (18.9 miles), from Batsto to CR 532 (16.6 miles), and from CR 532 to Ong (14 miles). Similarly, a thru-hike of the entire 50-mile trail could be planned, taking into account additional distances to campsites, all of which are off the trail.

NEARBY
Of course, you're in the middle of one of the most highly urbanized areas of the United States, so you're never very far from any services you might require. Hammonton, New Jersey, has a good selection of businesses. Atlantic City is only 27 miles away.

ADDITIONAL INFORMATION
For more information, visit the State of New Jersey's Department of Environmental Protection at state.nj.us/dep/parksandforests. You may also contact the Bass River State Forest at 609-296-1114.

TRIP 30
HITTING THE HIGH NOTES

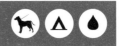

Location: Delaware Water Gap National Recreation Area, Stokes State Forest, and High Point State Park, New Jersey
Highlights: Rattlesnake Mountain, Mount Mohican, Sunrise Mountain, High Point
Distance: 44.1 miles one-way
Total Elevation Gain/Loss: 7,014 feet gain/6,220 feet loss
Trip Length: 3–6 days
Difficulty: Challenging
Recommended Maps and Other Resources:
- *Appalachian Trail Guide to New York-New Jersey*, 17th ed. Harpers Ferry, MD: Appalachian Trail Conservancy, 2011.
- National Park Service. *Delaware Water Gap.* nps.gov/dewa/ planyourvisit/upload/AT2012COLOR.pdf.
- USGS Quads: Stroudsburg, Portland, Bushkill, Flatbrookville, Branchville, and Point Jervis South.

This northbound section-hike on the Appalachian Trail (AT) will treat you to a jewel of a backpacking trip with one big vista after another. From glacial lakes like Sunfish Pond and Crater Lake to the big views from Rattlesnake and Sunrise mountains, you'll find yourself continually surprised and delighted by the beauty of the walk. And when you reach the monument to U.S. war dead standing atop High Point, with expansive views of Pennsylvania, New York, and New Jersey, you'll feel that you've completed a kind of pilgrimage. Few backcountry trips can boast of so dramatic a finish.

HIKE OVERVIEW

Following the northward track of the AT from where it enters New Jersey at the Delaware Water Gap, this trip follows the trail to High Point and the New York state line. Effectively, you'll walk from Pennsylvania to New York and cover almost two-thirds of the AT within New Jersey. From I-80 and the water gap, you'll climb up to the ridge of the Kittatinny Mountains and proceed north for 26 miles to Culvers Gap, passing glacial lakes and viewpoints including Mount Mohican and Rattlesnake Mountain. From the gap, you'll return to the ridgeline and make for High Point, first passing Sunrise Mountain and the rocky terrain near the Rutherford Shelter. With fair weather, expect to enjoy one grand view after another, but don't expect the ground to be easy. You may be in one of the most populated areas of the United States, but these miles along the AT are challenging. The footing is often rocky and treacherous, especially as you approach High Point.

In 2012, AMC legally challenged the National Park Service permit allowing construction of the Susquehanna to Roseland transmission line through the Delaware Water Gap National Recreation Area, but as of August 2013, the suit was unsuccessful. The National Park Service, however, will require the utility companies to provide $66 million in mitigation funding to offset the impact. Construction work in the area has begun and will continue through June 2015. Contact park headquarters or visit nps.gov/dewa/parkmgmt/power-line-updates .htm for a comprehensive list of temporary trail and facility closures.

HOW TO REACH THE TRAILHEAD

To Reach the Ending Trailhead. From Pennsylvania, head east on I-84. Take Exit 2 for Mountain Road, and then take a left on CR 55/Mountain Road. Continue south on this road for about 3.3 miles. As you cross the state line from New York into New Jersey, the name of the road changes to CR 519/Greenville Road. About 0.25 mile past the stateline, turn into the parking bay on the right (41° 19.760' N, 74° 38.594' W). The AT crosses CR 519 here.

To Reach the Starting Trailhead. Return to I-84, heading west to Exit 53 for Matamoras, Pennsylvania, and US 209. Follow US 209 south along the Delaware River, then take I-80 east. As you cross the river, you'll see blazes for the AT on the pedestrian walkway to the right. Take the first exit in New Jersey and park in the parking lot for the Kittatinny Point Visitor Center (40° 58.2077' N, 75° 7.7608' W).

OVERNIGHT OPTIONS

Backcountry camping along this stretch of the AT is regulated carefully, so it pays to know the rules before you go. So long as you're in the Delaware Water Gap National Recreation Area, backcountry camping is permitted if you are hiking for two or more consecutive days, but with a number of restrictions. You are limited to one night per campsite, ten people per campsite, and you must use stoves; fires are not allowed. You may not camp within 100 feet of a water source, within 0.5 mile of a road, within 200 feet of another party, or from 0.5 mile south of Blue Mountain Lake to 1 mile north of Crater Lake.

Once you are north of the recreation area, camping is only allowed near the five AT shelters. Campfires are still prohibited.

AMC's Mohican Outdoor Center (leave route at 8.67/1,117, center located at 41° 02.090' N, 75° 00.090' W). As you proceed along the AT, almost 9 miles north of the Water Gap, turn left on Camp Road. For a backpacker, this is the most luxurious place to stay on the trip. Not only are there cabins and rooms available in the lodge, but there is a camp store, showers, and, depending on the season, meals. The backcountry campsites are free for backpackers walking the trail. For more information, visit outdoors.org/lodging/mohican.

Backcountry Campsites along the Ridge of the Kittatinny There are three stretches where ridgeline camping is permitted in the recreation area: north of Catfish Pond Gap (9.5/1,449/41° 02.109' N, 74° 59.573' W), north of the Millbrook-Blairstown Road (14.4/1,502/41° 04.660' N, 74° 55.700' W), and just short of Rattlesnake Mountain (17.9/1,525/41° 07.085' N, 74° 53.276' W). As you walk through these areas, you'll spot many available sites, some of which have lovely views looking eastward. They tend to be dry, however, so bring your water in with you or plan on filling up at the water sources that bracket these areas.

AT Shelters North of the Delaware Water Gap Recreation Area Once you reach Stokes State Forest and High Point State Park, you'll need to stay either at shelters or in their immediate vicinity. There are a total of five shelters: Brinks Road (22.5/1,105/41° 09.194' N, 74° 50.266' W), Gren Anderson (29.5/1,300/41° 11.969' N, 74° 45.158' W), Mashipacong (35.2/1,435/41° 15.13' N, 74° 41.156' W), Rutherford (turn off at 38.1/1,440/41° 16.648' N, 74° 40.668' W), and High Point (turn off at 42.4/1,329, shelter at 41° 18.945' N, 74° 39.435' W). Brinks Road Shelter is located on an active forest road, so traffic noise could be a consideration; I also found that the water source was stagnant. The Gren Anderson, Rutherford, and High Point shelters each have water, but Rutherford is some distance (about 0.4 mile) off the AT.

HIKE DESCRIPTION

From the parking lot at the currently closed Kittatinny Point Visitor Center, follow the white blazes and walk east along I-80 until you see the overpass on the left. Pass beneath the bridge and walk back west along the highway until you see a day-hiker's parking lot on the left. The AT heads north from this parking lot, climbing gently along the left bank of Dunnfield Creek, which is quite picturesque along its lower reaches. The trail climbs for a total of 1,300 feet over a little more than 6 miles, but the path is well graded and is frequently traveled by day-hikers. Eventually, you'll reach a trail sign for Douglas Trail (3.41/1,286), which descends to the Worthington State Forest Campground.

DELAWARE WATER GAP NORTH

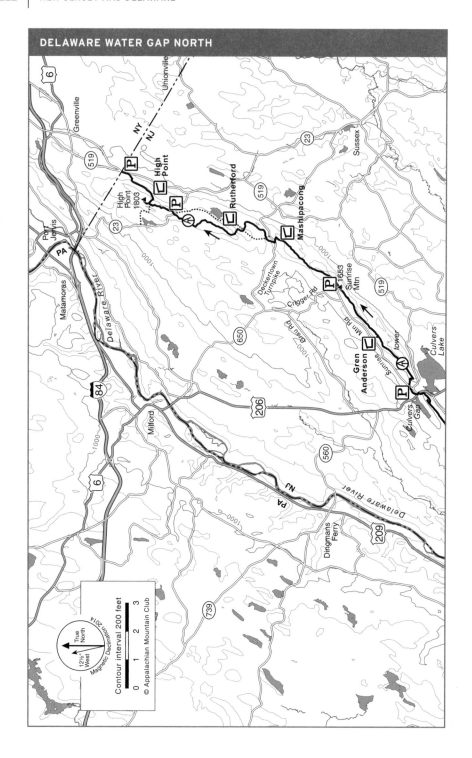

Contour interval 200 feet

True North

12½° West

Magnetic Declination 2014

© Appalachian Mountain Club

0   1   2   3

DELAWARE WATER GAP SOUTH

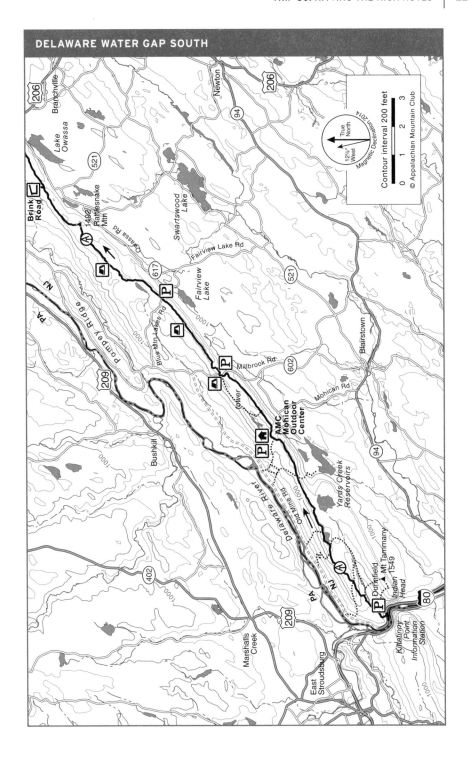

Note that at this point, you've not yet reached the Delaware Water Gap National Recreation Area and are within Worthington State Forest. The only backcountry camping is at the intersection of the AT with Douglas Trail.

In 4.1 miles, the AT reaches Sunfish Pond (1,392), one of New Jersey's seven natural wonders. Carved by the Wisconsin Glacier during the last ice age, this beautiful tarn is surrounded by steep, rocky shores and stands of mountain laurel and sheep laurel. The water of the pond is especially acidic, so only a few hardy species of fish can thrive there. The AT winds its way along the pond's rugged westward shore, passing several tempting little coves, but swimming and camping are prohibited.

From Sunfish Pond, the AT stays high up on the ridgeline and runs north to Mount Mohican (6.27/1,562). Superior views look to the northwest toward a bend in the Delaware River far below. From this prominence, the AT descends first to the intersection with Kaiser Trail on the left and then, somewhat more steeply, to Catfish Pond Gap and Camp Road (8.7/1,113). You'll also see red-blazed Coppermines Trail on the left. Just as you reach this road, you'll cross a small stream where you can refill your bottles. If you're planning to camp in the next section of trail, get water here, as the ridgeline will be dry until you reach Millbrook Road and Rattlesnake Spring, a little more than 3 miles ahead. (If you're bound for AMC's Mohican Outdoor Center, take a left on Camp Road and you'll be there in a quick spell.)

The AT climbs about 450 feet from Catfish Pond Gap to reach the ridgeline, immediately offering big views off to the east and flat spaces suitable for making camp. If night is falling, choose a spot, but the eastward-looking cliffs also become steeper as you go along and there is no shortage of campsites. The panorama shows off the contrast between the mountain forest and the densely populated east—you are, after all, fairly close to Manhattan.

The AT remains easy walking over the next 2 miles as it traces its way along the cliffs. The impressive views culminate when you reach the Catfish Fire Tower (10.9/1,551). The top of the tower is locked, but you can walk up the stairs to just beneath the top floor. From the tower, the AT descends to Rattlesnake Spring and Millbrook Road (11.8/1,239), flirting with a forest road as it goes. Though there are campsites here with easy access to water, they are quite close to the road, and they lack the views of the ridgeline campsites.

After crossing Milbrook Road (keep your eye out for a quick turn to the left), the AT rounds a glacial tarn and then reaches a gap where it climbs steeply to the right. It eventually reaches a power cut, which it follows past two towers. The trail then bends left and continues north for several miles of easy walking along the ridgeline. This section of the trail is dotted with campsites positioned to enjoy the views to the east. They are dry, but water is easily obtained at Millbrook Road to the south. This section ends at Blue Mountain Lakes Road (15.5/1,379), where there is a water pump.

Over the next few miles, the AT continues its northward ridge ramble, though the easiest walking is behind you. The trail soon grows rocky and even requires a little scrambling in places. At moments, the trail runs along slabby sections of ground that will test your rock-hopping abilities. Get used to this sort of footing because, if anything, the tread will become more fractured as you approach High Point. After crossing a flat stretch of forest, the AT scrambles over a rock wall to reach a view to the west. Pass a spur trail to Hemlock Pond and another to Buttermilk Falls (18.0/1,532). At 200 feet, these falls are New Jersey's highest. You can reach them by following the blue-blazed spur trail about 1.6 miles off the ridgeline. You'll also spot a nice site at the spur's intersection with the AT, if you're thinking of camping.

As it approaches Rattlesnake Mountain, the AT winds its way through a forested area and eventually reaches a gap where a footbridge crosses a creek. There's a campsite in this area, but even if you don't camp here, fill up your bottles. The next water source is at Brink Road Shelter just ahead, but I observed that the source was rather stagnant. The next sure water is at Gren Anderson Shelter, about 10 miles farther along.

After the campsite, the AT begins a short but steep climb to the top of Rattlesnake Mountain (18.8/1,557). The westward views of Pennsylvania from this summit are some of the trip's highlights.

When you reach Brink Road (22.7/1,163), you can turn left and walk about 0.2 mile to the shelter, or you can press onward. After about 3 miles of walking, you'll reach gorgeous views of Lake Owassa and Culvers Lake on your right. Ahead, you can see the line of mountains the AT is following. You should be able to spot the fire tower that stands atop the peak just beyond the gap. You'll be passing this point in about 3 miles.

Don't be so distracted by this view that you miss the AT, however. Just after the best views, a cairn marks where the AT takes a sharp rightward turn and begins descending with the ridgeline on the left and the lakes on the right (25.2/1,354). If you miss the turn, you'll eventually notice the absence of blazes—retrace your path until you find the cairn. The descent to Culvers Gap and US 206 is fairly steep. Once you've reached the road (26.3/926), you might think that the AT crosses the road and swings right. It doesn't—it swings left, crosses CR 636, and then heads north.

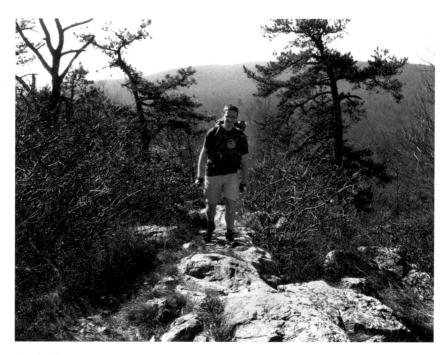

The footing along the AT in the Kittatinny Mountains can be rocky and treacherous, but the trail provides many attractive views as compensation.

The sounds of traffic in Culvers Gap will not likely entice you, but there are a few local businesses nearby, including a tavern and a convenience store. You could arrange a resupply here, if you wanted.

Once you're ready to proceed, pass an AT parking lot in the forest and then begin the 600-foot climb back up to the ridgeline. It's not terrifically difficult, by any means, but it will get your attention at the end of a long day. The good news is that, when you crest the ridge, you have a few miles of easy walking, first to the fire tower (28.3/1,508), where you may meet locals enjoying the fine views westward, and then to the Gren Anderson Shelter (located on a short spur trail to the left) and the creek that runs near it (29.3/1,310).

From the Gren Anderson Shelter, the AT follows a fairly even ridgeline until it reaches the summit of Sunrise Mountain (32.1/1,642). At the top, there is a large pavilion with views of the surrounding countryside. Even with High Point a few miles farther along, it's well worth pausing here to take in the sights.

The AT passes by the nearby parking lot and continues 3 miles along a sometimes slabby ridgeline to Mashipacong Shelter (35.3/1,425). From there, it crosses CR 650 and winds its way through the forest until it reaches the turnoff for Rutherford Shelter, which is 0.4 mile down in a basin (38.1/1,440). Although the trail is unrelentingly rocky from Mashipacong Shelter to High Point, the rockiest terrain is just north of this turnoff. Because this is the most rugged portion of the trail, you would do well to slow your pace. Several sections are almost as fractured and uneven as a lava field. In particular, you'll encounter one downward section of scrambling that merits particular care.

After a passing spur trail, the AT finally eases up, branches right away from the ridgeline, and brings you to the intersection with NJ 23, where there is parking lot and a ranger station (40.5/1,503). A short but rocky climb from NJ 23 will bring you back to the ridgeline, where you'll soon be able to see the obelisk commemorating U.S. war dead standing atop the 1,803-foot mountain. The AT will take you past an observation deck with excellent views of the obelisk (41.4/1,689), but to reach the memorial, you'll have to turn off on a blue-blazed spur trail that climbs to the summit (41.8/1,803). The views of Pennsylvania, New Jersey, and New York are well worth the effort. Savor, especially, the southward view looking back over your journey, as this is truly the "high point" of the trip.

From the memorial, descend to the AT, turn east (or left), and begin the walk that winds its way around High Point and soon turns east to run parallel to the New York state line. The initial descent is sharp and rocky, but after you pass the turnoff for the High Point Shelter, the trail relents to easy walking through increasingly agricultural land. The trail dips down to CR 519, where your shuttle vehicle is waiting (43.6/1,105). Walk out and back about a quarter-mile north to cross the state line, if you're interested in the bragging rights (44.1/1,105).

OTHER OPTIONS

If you add many more miles to the New Jersey section of the AT, you'll very rapidly be closing in on section-hiking the whole of the trail in the state. Such an undertaking is beyond the scope of this book, but you could accomplish it by positioning the northernmost vehicle at Greenwood Lake.

Of course, there is quite a bit more hiking to be done in the Delaware Water Gap itself, and you could also expand the hike by adding some of the scenic spur trails that branch off the AT. For one option, climb to the summit of the 1,250-feet Mount Tammany for classic views of the Delaware River. Take Red Dot (Tammany) Trail from the parking lot where the AT begins to ascend Dunnfield Creek to reach the Indian Head scenic view in about 1.5 miles of climbing. Descend 2.5 miles down Blue Dot Trail to rejoin the AT.

To shorten the trip, break it into two weekend hikes by placing a vehicle at Culvers Gap and hike from I-80 to Sunfish Pond, then Rattlesnake Mountain on the second day. The northern section of the trip could also be done in a weekend, northbound, by hiking in to Gren Andersen Shelter on a Friday, to Rutherford Shelter on Saturday, and finishing up with High Point on Sunday. A similar trip could be walked southbound using High Point Shelter.

NEARBY

You'll see many local businesses as you drive along US 209. Milford, Pennsylvania, is an especially picturesque little town.

ADDITIONAL INFORMATION

You may call the Delaware Water Gap National Recreation Area at 570-426-2451, the Worthington State Forest at 908-841-9575, the Stokes State Forest 973-948-3820, and High Point State Park at 973-875-4800 for more information. For emergencies, call 800-543-4295, 24 hours a day. The Water Gap is not an especially isolated area—my phone had reception for the entire trip.

RESOURCES

ONLINE

We in the Mid-Atlantic benefit from several excellent online resources. Though both tend to focus on day hikes, they also list backpacking trips. And, of course, a backpacking trip can often be made by connecting the dots between several day hikes in a given area.

- HikingUpward.com
- MidAtlanticHikes.com

THE POTOMAC APPALACHIAN TRAIL CLUB (PATC)

PATC's publications are indispensable resources for hiking in the region. Their maps and books may often be found in outdoors stores, but can also be purchased online at patc.net. (Maps 1-13 cover the Appalachian Trail from Virginia to Pennsylvania; Maps G, H, and F cover Massanutten Mountain and Great North Mountain.)

- Palatini, Glenn. *Guide to the Great North Mountain Trail.* Vienna, VA: PATC. 2008.
- PATC. *Appalachian Trail Guide Book #6 (Maryland and N. Virginia),* 17th ed., Vienna, VA: PATC. 2008.
- PATC. *Appalachian Trail Guide Book #7 (Shenandoah NP and Side Trails),* 14th ed., Vienna, VA: PATC. 2012.
- PATC. *Circuit Hikes in Shenandoah National Park*, 17th ed., Vienna, VA: PATC. 2013.
- PATC. *Circuit Hikes in Virginia, West Virginia, Maryland, and Pennsylvania*, 9th ed., Vienna, VA: PATC. 2013.
- PATC. *Guide to Massanutten Mountain Hiking Trails*, 5th ed., Vienna, VA: PATC. 2013.
- PATC. *The Potomac Appalachian Trail Club's Cabins.* Vienna, VA: PATC. 2013.

Appalachian Trail Guides

Of course, the Appalachian Trail is one of the great features of the region for hikers. There is no shortage of books published on this great American footpath, but I recommend that serious hikers acquire the Appalachian Trail Conservancy's guides for the region. These books ship with excellent maps focused on the AT and they are easily found for purchase online.

- Chazin, Daniel D. *Appalachian Trail Guide to New York-New Jersey*, 17th ed. Harpers Ferry, WV: Appalachian Trail Conservancy. 2010.
- Dillon, Tom. *Appalachian Trail Guide to Southwest Virginia*, 5th ed. Harpers Ferry, WV: Appalachian Trail Conservancy. 2010.
- Graf, Irma. *Appalachian Trail Guide to Central Virginia*, 2nd ed. Harpers Ferry, WV: Appalachian Trail Conservancy. 2010.

WEST VIRGINIA

These books are easier to find online at the sites listed than other stores, but are certainly worth seeking out.

- deHart, Alan and Bruce Sundquist. *Monongahela National Forest Hiking Guide*, 8th ed. West Virginia Highlands Conservancy. [You can obtain this book at wvhighlands.org either in paper or on a CD. The maps that come with the CD are especially useful.]
- Juskelis, Michael V. *The Mid-Atlantic Hiker's Guide: West Virginia*. Spring Mills, PA: Scott Adams Enterprises. 2013. [Available at pahikes.com]

PENNSYLVANIA

Often, for Pennsylvania trails, you'll want to acquire the individual books and maps published by the local trail clubs. These are very handy and are listed in the relevant chapters. Pahikes.com stocks a good array of them. Pine Creek Outfitters also stocks many of these books (pinecrk.com, 570-724-3003). Always check out what Pennsylvania's Department of Conservation and Natural Resources has to offer. Not only are there maps online (dcnr.state.pa.us/forestry/recreation/hiking/stateforesttrails/), but a quick phone call will often get you a free, high-quality map printed on water-resistant paper. Two state-specific, must-have additions follow.

- Mitchell, Jeff. *Backpacking Pennsylvania: 37 Great Hikes*. Mechanicsburg, PA: Stackpole Books. 2005.
- Keystone Trails Association. *Pennsylvania Hiking Trails*, ed. Ben Cramer. Mechanicsburg, PA: Stackpole Books. 2008

NEW YORK AND NEW JERSEY

Just as PATC's resources are some of the best available for the southern reaches of the Mid-Atlantic, the publications of the Adirondack Mountain Club (adk. org) are your go-to resources for the Catskills and the Adirondacks. If you're hiking closer to the city, you'll want to scope out the maps sold by the New York-New Jersey Trail Conference (nynjtc.org).

Books

- Adirondack Mountain Club. *High Peaks Trails*, 14th ed., eds. Tony Goodwin and David Tomas-Train. Lake George, NY: Adirondack Mountain Club. 2012.

Maps

- Adirondack Mountain Club. *Trails Illustrated Map 742: Lake Placid/High Peaks*. Evergreen, CO: National Geographic Maps and Adirondack Mountain Club. 2012.
- Kick, Peter. *Catskill Mountain Guide*, 3e. Boston, MA: Appalachian Mountain Club. 2014.
- New York-New Jersey Trail Conference. *Catskill Trails*, 10th ed. Mahwah, NJ: New York-New Jersey Trail Conference. 2013.
- New York-New Jersey Trail Conference. *Harriman-Bear Mountain Trails*, 15th ed. Mahwah, NJ: New York-New Jersey Trail Conference. 2013.

DELAWARE AND THE DELMARVA PENINSULA

Though your opportunities for backpacking in this area are limited, there is at least one guide you should acquire.

- Abercrombie, Jay. *Weekend Walks on the Delmarva Peninsula: Walks and Hikes in Delaware and the Eastern Shore of Maryland and Virginia*, 2nd ed. Woodstock, VT: Countryman Press. 2006

INDEX

A

Adirondack Forest Preserve, xii–xv, xxxi, 150–172
Adirondack Loj, 161, 165
Adirondack Shelters, MD, 175
Allegheny Front Trail (AFT), xii–xiii, xxxviii, 113–120
alpine zone, xxxvii
Annapolis Rocks, 197–198, 200–201
Anthony Wayne Recreation Area, 138
Appalachian balds, xxxvii
Appalachian Mountain Club (AMC), 241, 243, 245–246
Appalachian Trail
guidebooks, 230
in Maryland, xiv–xv, xxxii, 190–206
in New Jersey, xxxiii, 219–228
in New York, xxxi, 138–141
in Pennsylvania, xxx, 121–126
in Virginia, 14–22, 24–29, 44–46, 49–56
Appalachian Trail Conservancy (ATC), 196, 230
Assateague, xiv–xv, xxxvi, 182–189
Assateague Island National Seashore, xiv–xv, xxxii, 182–189
Ausable River, 156, 162
author's favorites, xviii
Avalanche Lake, xxxii, 158, 165

B

backpacks, xlvii–xlviii
Back TO NAture Trail (BATONA), xiv–xv, 213–218
baldcypress trees, xxxvi, 208, 211
Bald Peak, NY, 171
barrier islands, xxxvi, 183, 188
Bass River State Park, 213–214, 216
beach trips, 182–189
Bear Den Mountain, 153
Bear Mountain, xii–xiii, xxxi, 138–142
Bear Run Nature Preserve, xii–xiii, 92–98
bears, black, xliii
Beaver Meadow Falls, 150, 156
berries, xlii, 72, 169
Big Flat Mountain, 52
Big Run, x–xi, 49–56
Big Schloss, 5, 84, 88–89
Birch Run Shelter, 123
birdwatching, recommended spots, 182, 208
Black Forest Trail (BFT), xii–xiii, 106–112
Black Moshannon State Park, 113–120
Black Rock, NY, 197, 201
Blackrock, VA, 49–51, 54–55
Blackrock Hut, 51–52
Brinks Road Shelter, 221
Brothers, The, 158, 166
Brown Mountain, 49, 53–54
Buttonwood Hill Camp, 216
Buzzard Rocks, 34, 36, 39

C

Caledonia State Park, xii–xiii, 121–126
camping, best sites for, xvi. *See also* individual trip descriptions
Canadian boreal forests, xxxvi–xxxvii
Catawba Mountain Shelter, 15
Catawba River, 14
Catoctin Mountain, xxxii
Cacotin Trail (CT), xiv–xv, 197–206
Cat Rock, 197–198, 204
Catskill Forest Preserve, xii–xiii, xxxi, 143–149
Cedar Run, 40, 43–44
Chimney Rock, 197–198, 204

Chimney Top, 78, 81–83
Chincoteague, VA, 189
Churchville, VA, 13
clothing, li–liii
C&O Canal, xiv–xv, 174–181
conservation, xxxvii–xxxviii
    Leave No Trace principles, lvii–lviii
cooking gear, xlviii–xlix
Corbin Cabin, 43
Cowall Shelter, 200
Crampton Gap Shelter, 191
Cross Fork, PA, 135
Cumberland, MD, 181
Cunningham Falls, 198, 202–203

D
Dahlgren Backpacker Campground, 191, 193
Damascus, VA, 30
day hikes, xvi
Delaware, trips in, xiv–xv, xxxii–xxxiii,
    208–212
    hiking guidebooks, 231
Delaware Water Gap, xiv–xv, xxxiii, 219–228
Delaware Water Gap National Recreation
    Area, xiv–xv, 219–228
Devil's Acre Lean-to, 146
Devil's Alley campsite, 175
Devil's Path, xii–xiii, xxxi, 143–149
Devil's Tombstone Campground, 146
Dial Mountain, 153
Diamond Notch Falls, 143, 146, 148
Dix Mountain Wilderness, xii–xiii, 150–157
Dolly Sods, x–xi, xxx, 58–64
Doyles River, 49, 52
Doyles River Cabin, 50
Dragon's Tooth, 14, 16, 18–22

E
Ed Garvey Shelter, 193
The Egg, NY, 142
electronics, liv–lv
Elizabeth Furnace Campground, 36
epic adventures, xviii

F
Fallingwater, 98
Fifteenmile Creek, 174, 177, 179
Fish Hawk Cliffs, 150–151, 155
fishing, xvii
Flatrock Plains, 72–73, 75
food, xlix
footwear, liii
fracking, xxxvii–xxxviii

Frederick, MD, 206
Front Royal, VA, 39
Furnace Mountain, 54

G
Gambrill State Park, xiv–xv, 197–206
Gathland State Park, 190, 193–194, 196
gear, xliv–lvi
    backpacks, xlvii–xlviii
    clothing, li–liii
    cooking gear, xlviii–xlix
    electronics, liv–lv
    food, xlix
    footwear, liii
    hygiene, l–li
    shelter considerations, xlv–xlvi
    sleeping considerations, xlvi–xlvii
    water, drinking, l
    weight considerations, lv–lvi
George Washington and Jefferson National
    Forests, x–xiii, 2–39, 84–90
Gettysburg, PA, 126
Giant Mountain, 168–169, 171
Giant Mountain Wilderness, xiv–xv, 168–172
Giardia, xliv
Godfrey Bridge Family Camp, 216
Grayson Highlands, x–xi, 24–30
Great North Mountain, WV, 84, 88–89
Great Traverse (Adirondacks), 166
Greenbriar State Park, xiv–xv, 190–196
Green Mountain, WV, 69
Green Ridge State Forest, xiv–xv, xxxii,
    174–181
Gren Anderson Shelter, 221
Grindstone Campground, 24, 26–27, 30
Grindstone Mountain, 9–10

H
Hagerstown, MD, 181
Halfmoon Mountain, 84–85, 87–88
Hammonton, NJ, 218
Harpers Ferry, WV, xxxv, 190–196
Harriman State Park, xii–xiii, xxxi, 138–142
Hawksbill Mountain, xxix, 40, 43–45
Heart Lake, 158, 161, 165–166
heatstroke, xli
Hemlock Mountain, 109
Highlands Coalition, xxxviii
High Peaks Region (Adirondacks, NY),
    xiv–xv, 150–172
High Point, xiv–xv, 219–228
High Point Shelter, 221

High Point State Park, 219, 221
  hiking guidebooks, 229–231
Hog Rock, 197–198, 202, 204
Hozack Hollow, 121
huckleberries, xlii
Hughes River, 46
Hunter Mountain, 145–146, 148
hygiene, l–li
hypothermia, xl–xli

I

Indian Head Mountain, 146, 150, 155
insects, xliii

J

Jefferson National Forest. See George
  Washington and Jefferson National
  Forests
Johns Brook Lodge, 159, 161, 163
Jones Run, 49, 52

K

Keene, NY, 157, 166, 172
Kennedy Peak, 31, 37
Kerns Mountain, 34, 38
Keystone Trails Association, 113, 230
kids, trips good for, xviii
Kittatinny Mountains, xxxiii

L

Lake Colden, xxxii, 158–161, 164–165
Lake Placid, NY, 157, 166, 172
lakes and ponds, hikes involving, xvii
Lamberts Meadow Shelter, 15
Laurel, DE, 210
Leave No Trace principles, lvii–lviii
less traveled trips, xviii
Little Crease Shelter, 35
Little Fort Recreation Area, 35
Loft Mountain Campground, 50, 52
Long Mountain, WV, 84–85, 87
Long Path, 142, 148
Long Pine Run Reservoir, 121, 124–125
Lookout Mountain, 9–10
Lyman Run State Park, 127, 131
Lyme disease, xliii

M

Manor Area Campground, 200
maps, liv
locator map, iv
Maryland, trips in, xiv–xv, xxxii, 173–206
Maryland Blue Ridge, xiv–xv, 190–197

Maryland Heights, 190, 195–196
Mary Louise Pond, 168–169, 171
Mashipacong Shelter, 221
Massanutten Mountain, x–xi, xxix, 31–39
McAfee Knob, 14–18
Michaux State Forest, xii–xiii, 121–126
Milford, PA, 228
Mink Hollow Shelter, 145–146
Mohican Outdoor Center, 221
Monongahela National Forest, x–xiii, 58–83
Moorefield, WV, 77
Moshannon Creek, 116
Moshannon State Forest, xii–xiii, 113–120
Mount Colvin, 155
Mount Marcy, 158
Mount Mohican, 219, 224
Mount Robertson, 47
Mount Rogers, 24, 26–27
Mount Rogers Recreation Area, 24–30
Mount Tammany, 227
Mount Zion Road Adirondacks Shelter, MD, 200

N

natural history, xxxvi–xxxvii
New Jersey, trips in, xiv–xv, xxxii–xxxiii,
  213–228
  hiking guidebooks, 231
New York, trips in, xii–xv, xxxi–xxxii,
  137–172
  hiking guidebooks, 231
Noonmark Mountain, 153
northern hardwood forests, xxxvi
North Fork Mountain, WV, xii–xiii, 78–83
North Mountain, VA, 14–15, 18–20
North River, VA, 6, 9–10

O

Ohiopyle, PA, 98
old-growth forest, 6
Old Rag Mountain, x–xi, 40–48
Ole Bull State Park, 127, 130, 132, 135
online resources, 229
Opalescent River, 159, 164
Ore Bed Shelter, 159
Otter Creek Wilderness, x–xi, xxx, 65–71
Overlook Shelter, 145
Owens Creek Campground, 200

P

Paw Paw Tunnel, xxxii, 174–175, 179
Paw Paw Tunnel Campground, 175, 178
Pennsylvania, trips in, xii–xiii, xxx–xxxi,
  91–136
hiking guidebooks, 230

Pennsylvania Blue Ridge, xii–xiii, 121–126
Pennsylvania Highlands Trail Network,
  xxxviii
Petersburg, WV, 77
piedmont forests, xxxvi
Pine Barrens, xxxvi, 213–218
Pine Creek Gorge, 99, 102–104, 106, 111
Pinelands National Preserve, xiv–xv, 213–218
plant hazards, xlii
Plateau Mountain, NY, 147
poison ivy, xlii
Potomac Appalachian Trail Club (PATC), 42,
  50, 125, 229
Potomac River, 174–181, 194–196
Powell Mountain, 38
Purslane Run campsite, 175

Q
Quarry Gap Shelter, 123

R
Ramseys Draft Wilderness, x–xi, 6–13
Rattlesnake Mountain, 219, 221, 225
Raven Rock, 197, 200, 202
Raven Rock Shelter, 200
Roanoke, VA, 22
Roaring Plains, xii–xiii, 72–77
Rock Spring Hut, 41
Rocky Knob, xii–xiii, 121–126
Rocky Mountain, VA, 53
Rocky Ridge Peak, 168, 171
Rocky Run Shelter, 191
Rutherford Shelter, 221

S
safety tips, xxxix–xl
Saint Anne's Peak, 148
Salisbury, MD, 212
Saranac Lake, NY, 172
Seaford, DE, 212
seasons, xxxiv–xxxvi
Seneca Rocks, WV, 71, 83
Shavers Mountain, 68
Shawangunk mountains, xxxi
shelter considerations, xlv–xlvi
Shenandoah National Park, x–xi, xxix, 40–56
  camping regulations in, 41
Shenandoah River, 31, 34
Short Mountain, VA, 34, 38
Signal Knob, 31, 34–35, 38
sleeping considerations, xlvi–xlvii
small mammals, xliii–xliv
Sorel Ridge campsite, 175
South Shore Campground, 214

Stickpile Hill campsite, 175
stinging nettle, xlii
Stokes State Forest, 219, 221
Stony Man, 40, 44–45
Sugarloaf Mountain, NY, 147
sunburn, xlii
Sunfish Pond, 219, 224
Sunrise Mountain, 219–220, 226
Susquehannock State Forest, xii–xiii, 127–136
Susquehannock Trail System, xii–xiii, xxxviii,
  127–136
swimming holes, xvi, xxxv. *See also* waterfalls
  in Maryland, 179
  in New York, 146, 148
  in Pennsylvania, 108, 134
  in Virginia, 10, 43, 49, 53, 55
  in West Virginia, 59, 65, 68–70

T
tarps, xlv–xlvi
tents, xlv–xlvi
Thomas Knob Shelter, 26
Three Top Mountain, 34, 38
Tiadaghton State Forest, xii–xiii, 106–112
Tibbet Knob, x–xi, 2–5, 84–85, 87–88
ticks, xxxv, xliii
Tinker Cliffs, 14–18, 22
Tioga State Forest, xii–xiii, 99–105
Trap Pond, xiv–xv, xxxii, xxxvi, 208–212
Trap Pond State Park, xiv–xv, 208–212
Trayfoot Mountain, 54–55
Triple Crown, x–xi, 14–23
trip planning, xxxix–lvi
Trout Run Valley, xii–xiii, 84–90
Tuscarora Trail, xxx, 89
Twin Mountain, NY, 147

U
unusual forests, xvi

V
views, big, xvii
Virginia, hikes in, x–xi, xxix–xxx, 1–56

W
Waonaze Peak, 38
water, drinking, l
water crossings, xli–xlii
Waterfall Mountain, 38
waterfalls, xvii. *See also* swimming holes
  in Maryland, 202–203
  in New York, 146, 156, 172
  in Pennsylvania, 110

in Virginia, 40, 49, 52, 59
in West Virginia, 62, 65, 70
weight considerations, lv–lvi
Wellsboro, PA, 105
West Kill Mountain, 148
West Mountain, NY, 138–140
West Mountain Shelter, 139–140
West Rim Trail (WRT), xii–xiii, xxxvii, 99–105
West Virginia, trips in, x–xiii, xxx, 57–90
hiking guidebooks, 230
West Virginia Highlands Conservancy, 230
wetlands, xxxvi, 208–212
Weverton Cliffs, 190, 194
White Rocks, xxxii, 190, 194
wildflowers, xviii, xxxv, 24
wildlife, xlii–xliv
recommended spots for encountering, 127, 178, 182, 188, 208
Wild Oak Trail, x–xi, 6–13
Williamsport, PA, 112, 135
Wise Shelter, 26
Wolf Gap Campground, 3
Woodstock, NY, 149
Woodstock, VA, 5, 89
Wright, Frank Lloyd, 98

Y
Yard Mountain, 165
Youghioheny River, 92, 96

ABOUT THE AUTHOR

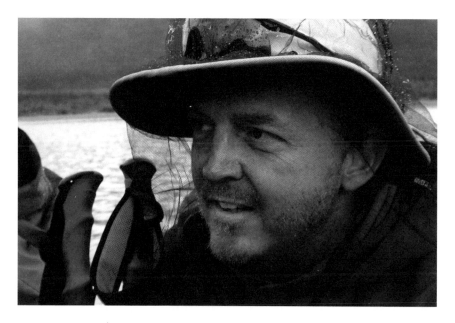

MICHAEL MARTIN is a lifelong backpacker and outdoorsman. He grew up on the trails in Texas, Arkansas, New Mexico, and Colorado, and points farther west; more recently, he has piled on several thousand miles (and a few hundred nights) in the Mid-Atlantic. His more exotic trips have taken him to Sweden, France, Nepal, Peru, and Iceland, where he completed a north-south crossing of the island—his most ambitious trip to date. He leads, organizes, and teaches for the DC UL Backpacking group. When he's not on the trail, or plotting new ways to sneak away and get on the trail, he's often writing, learning how to make his camera work, or trying to limber up his rusty video-gaming skills. His more permanent dwelling is Old Town Alexandria, with his wife Laura Lewellyn (Fancy Pants) and his Yorkshire terrier Ginger.

Appalachian Mountain Club

Founded in 1876, AMC is the nation's oldest outdoor recreation and conservation organization. AMC promotes the protection, enjoyment, and understanding of the mountains, forests, waters, and trails of the Northeast outdoors.

People

We are more than 150,000 members, advocates, and supporters, including 12 local chapters, more than 16,000 volunteers, and over 450 full-time and seasonal staff. Our chapters reach from Maine to Washington, D.C.

Outdoor Adventure and Fun

We offer more than 8,000 trips each year, from local chapter activities to adventure travel worldwide, for every ability level and outdoor interest— from hiking and climbing to paddling, snowshoeing, and skiing.

Great Places to Stay

We host more than 150,000 guests each year at our AMC lodges, huts, camps, shelters, and campgrounds. Each AMC destination is a model for environmental education and stewardship.

Opportunities for Learning

We teach people skills to safely enjoy the outdoors and to care for the natural world around us through programs for children, teens, and adults, as well as outdoor leadership training.

Caring for Trails

We maintain more than 1,800 miles of trails throughout the Northeast, including nearly 350 miles of the Appalachian Trail in five states.

Protecting Wild Places

We advocate for land and riverway conservation, monitor air quality, research climate change, and work to protect alpine and forest ecosystems throughout the Northern Forest and Mid-Atlantic Highlands regions.

Engaging the Public

We seek to educate and inform our own members and an additional 2 million people annually through the media, AMC Books, our website, our White Mountain visitor centers, and AMC destinations.

Join Us!

Members meet other like-minded people and support our mission while enjoying great AMC programs, our award-winning *AMC Outdoors* magazine, and special discounts. Visit outdoors.org or call 800-372-1758 for more information.

APPALACHIAN MOUNTAIN CLUB
Recreation • Education • Conservation
outdoors.org

AMC IN THE MID-ATLANTIC

EACH YEAR, AMC'S DELAWARE VALLEY, MOHAWK HUDSON, New York/New Jersey, and Washington, D.C. chapters offer thousands of outdoor activities including hiking, backpacking, bicycling, paddling, and climbing trips, as well as social, family, and young member programs. Members also maintain local trails, lead outdoor skills workshops, and promote stewardship of the region's natural resources. To view a list of AMC activities in the Mid-Atlantic and across the Northeast, visit activities.outdoors.org.

AMC is a leader of the Highlands Coalition, which works to secure funding for land conservation funding in the four-state Highlands region of Connecticut, New York, New Jersey, and Pennsylvania. It is also active in addressing energy development projects and impact public lands, and is leading the effort to establish the Pennsylvania Highlands Trail Network. To learn more about AMC's conservation work in the Highlands, visit outdoors.org/conservation/wherewework/highlands/index.cfm

AMC BOOK UPDATES

AMC BOOKS STRIVES TO KEEP OUR GUIDEBOOKS AS UP-TO-DATE as possible to help you plan safe and enjoyable adventures. If after publishing a book we learn that trails have been relocated or route or contact information has changed, we will post the updated information online. Before you hit the trail, check for updates at outdoors.org/bookupdates.

While hiking, if you notice discrepancies with the trip description or map, or if you find any other errors in the book, please let us know by submitting them to amcbookupdates@outdoors.org or in writing to Books Editor, c/o AMC, 5 Joy Street, Boston, MA 02108. We will verify all submissions and post key updates each month. AMC Books is dedicated to being a recognized leader in outdoor publishing. Thank you for your participation.

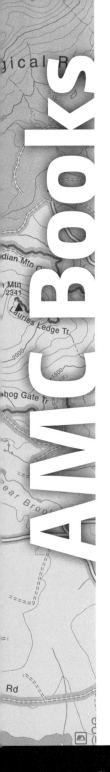

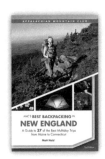

AMC's Best Backpacking in New England, 2nd Edition

Matt Heid

Explore the region's wildest trails in 37 overnight trips, from maritime delights of Cape Cod's Sandy Neck and Maine's Cutler Coast, to the wild forests of Monroe State Forest in Massachusetts and Vermont's Glastenbury Mountain Wilderness, to classic backpacking pilgrimages through the 100-Mile Wilderness and across the Presidential Range.

$19.95 • 978-1-934028-90-2

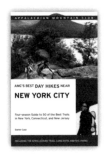

AMC's Best Day Hikes Near New York City

Daniel Case

Enjoy 50 of the best year-round excursions in New York, Connecticut, and northern New Jersey. Hike the Palisades Interstate Park, explore the Shawangunk Grasslands National Wildlife Refuge, discover the Paugussett State Forest, or even ramble through Central Park from end to end.

$18.95 • 978-1-934028-38-4

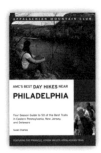

AMC's Best Day Hikes Near Philadelphia

Susan Charkes

Tour 50 of the best hikes in Eastern Pennsylvania, New Jersey, and Delaware year-round. Walk through historic Valley Forge, discover the beautiful French Creek State Park, see the Pinnacle's spectacular views, and visit New Jersey's famed Pine Barrens.

$18.95 • 978-1-934028-33-9

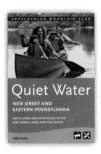

Quiet Water New Jersey and Eastern Pennsylvania

Kathy Kenley

Great for families, anglers, and canoeists and kayakers of all abilities, this guide features 80 trips, covering the best calm water paddling in the region. Paddle through Lake Aeroflex and connecting ponds, spot wildlife in South Jersey's Great Bay, or discover the beautiful French Creek State Park on water.

$19.95 • 978-1-934028-34-6

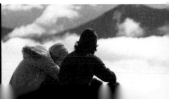